Additional Parenting Books From the American Academy of Pediatrics

Caring for Your Baby and Young Child: Birth to Age 5
(English and Spanish)

Heading Home With Your Newborn:
From Birth to Reality

Mommy Calls: Dr. Tanya Answers Parents' Top 101 Questions

DATE DUE ild

Su..)nes

Raising Twins: From Pregnancy to Preschool

Your Baby's First Year
(English and Spanish)

New Mother's Guide to Breastfeeding
(English and Spanish)

Food Fights: Winning the Nutritional Challenges of Parenthood
Armed With Insight, Humor, and a Bottle of Ketchup

A Parent's Guide to Childhood Obesity: A Road Map to Health

Guide to Your Child's Nutrition

ADHD: A Complete and Authoritative Guide

Waking Up Dry: A Guide to Help Children Overcome Bedwetting

A Parent's Guide to Building Resilience in Children and Teens:
Giving Your Child Roots and Wings

Sports Success R$_x$! Your Child's Prescription for the Best Experience

Less Stress, More Success: A New Approach to Guiding Your Teen
Through College Admissions and Beyond

Mental Health, Naturally: The Family Guide to Holistic Care
for a Healthy Mind and Body

Caring for Your School-Age Child:
Ages 5 to 12

Caring for Your Teenager

Guide to Toilet Training
(English and Spanish)

CyberSafe: Protecting and Empowering Kids in the Digital World
of Texting, Gaming, and Social Media

**For more information, please visit the official AAP Web site for parents,
www.HealthyChildren.org/bookstore.**

ALLERGIES AND ASTHMA

2ND EDITION

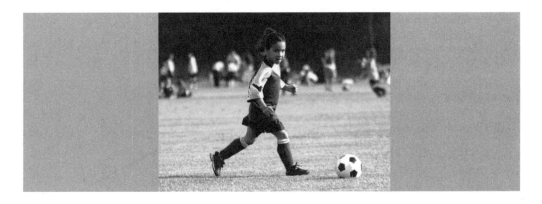

What Every Parent Needs to Know

MICHAEL J. WELCH, MD, FAAAAI, FAAP, CPI

EDITOR IN CHIEF

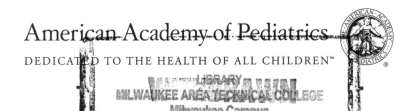

American Academy of Pediatrics

DEDICATED TO THE HEALTH OF ALL CHILDREN™

American Academy of Pediatrics Department of Marketing and Publications Staff

Director, Department of Marketing and Publications
Maureen DeRosa, MPA

Director, Division of Product Development
Mark Grimes

Manager, Consumer Publishing
Carolyn Kolbaba

Coordinator, Product Development
Holly Kaminski

Director, Division of Publishing and Production Services
Sandi King, MS

Editorial Specialist
Jason Crase

Print Production Specialist
Shannan Martin

Manager, Art Direction and Production
Linda Diamond

Director, Division of Marketing and Sales
Kevin Tuley

Manager, Consumer Product Marketing
Kathleen Juhl

Published by the American Academy of Pediatrics
141 Northwest Point Blvd, Elk Grove Village, IL 60007-1019
847/434-4000
Fax: 847/434-8000
www.aap.org

Cover design by Daniel Rembert
Book design by Linda Diamond
Illustrations by Graphic World

Second Edition—2011
First Edition—© 2000 as *Guide to Your Child's Allergies and Asthma: Breathing Easy
and Bringing Up Healthy, Active Children*

Library of Congress Control Number: 2010900143
ISBN: 978-1-58110-445-5

What People Are Saying

Ever wish you could sit down and spend hours asking your pediatrician every question you never remember to ask at appointments? Read this practical, must-have resource for all parents of children with allergies and asthma—and you'll have your answers.

Nancy Sander
President and Founder, Allergy & Asthma Network Mothers of Asthmatics

A valuable and highly usable addition to the field of asthma and allergy management.

Bill McLin
President and CEO, Asthma and Allergy Foundation of America

This excellent book provides parents with the facts, the concepts, and the approach they need to care for their child with allergies or asthma. This second edition is a joy to read. It flows smoothly and covers the important issues with ample detail.

Thomas F. Plaut, MD, FAAP
Director, Asthma Consultants, and author, *One Minute Asthma: What You Need to Know*

This book is an excellent resource. Parents and grandparents of children with allergic diseases will find the same basic principles for diagnosing and treating these conditions as their physicians, but in an easy-to-read style. I found the "Asthma Facts and Fables" a particularly nice touch.

Jeffrey R. Stokes, MD, FAAAAI, FACAAI
Associate Professor, Creighton University Medical Center, and spokesperson,
American Academy of Allergy, Asthma & Immunology

If you want a book that describes unproven therapies that may not work, stay away. But if you want a detailed and comprehensive book that describes state-of-the-art understanding and approaches to asthma and allergies in children written by the leading experts in the field, this book is essential reading. If you want to know what you should ask and what you should expect from your doctor when you have a child with asthma and/or allergies—this book is for you. If you want to know both the natural approaches that are documented to work and how to get the most out of medications, then this book is for you.

Harold J. Farber, MD, MSPH, FAAP
Associate Professor of Pediatrics, Pulmonary Section, Baylor College of Medicine;
author of *Control Your Child's Asthma: A Breakthrough Program for the Treatment and Management of Childhood Asthma*; and editor of *Pediatric Allergy, Immunology, and Pulmonology*

Acknowledgments

Editor in Chief
Michael J. Welch, MD, FAAAAI, FAAP, CPI

American Academy of Pediatrics Board of Directors Reviewer
Kenneth E. Matthews, MD, FAAP

Reviewers/Contributors
Stuart Abramson, MD, FAAAAI, FAAP
Sami Labib Bahna, MD, FAAAAI, FAAP
A. Wesley Burks, MD, FAAAAI, FAAP
Bradley E. Chipps, MD, PhD, FAAAAI, FAAP
John Duplantier, MD, FAAAAI, FAAP
Howard Eigen, MD, FAAP
Mary Beth Fasano, MD, FAAAAI, FAAP
Alan Goldsobel, MD, FAAAAI, FAAP
Douglas N. Homnick, MD, MPH, FAAP
Russell Hopp, DO, FAAAAI, FAAP
Julie Pamela Katkin, MD, FAAP
John Kelso, MD, FAAAAI, FAAP
Mitchell Ross Lester, MD, FAAAAI, FAAP
Todd A. Mahr, MD, FAAAAI, FAAP
Elizabeth C. Matsui, MD, FAAAAI, FAAP
Susanna A. McColley, MD, FAAP
Sai Nimmagadda, MD, FAAAAI, FAAP
Lynda Catherine Schneider, MD, FAAAAI, FAAP
Scott Howard Sicherer, MD, FAAAAI, FAAP
Miles M. Weinberger, MD, FAAP
Paul Victor Williams, MD, FAAAAI, FAAP
Robert Alan Wood, MD, FAAAAI

Additional Assistance
Debra L. Burrowes, MHA
Laura Laskosz, MPH

Writer
Winnie Yu

To all the people who recognize that children are our greatest inspiration in the present and our greatest hope for the future.

From the Editor in Chief

To the many children out there who are

The sneezers and wheezers
The sniffers and whiffers

The scratchers and rashers
The coughers and hackers

The itchers and twitchers
The snorers and blowers

Relief is in sight
In the pages just right

Hoping a look at this book
Was all that it took.

—MJW

Table of Contents

Please Note

The information contained in this book is intended to complement, not substitute for, the advice of your child's pediatrician. Before starting any medical treatment or program, you should consult with your child's pediatrician, who can discuss your child's individual needs and counsel you about symptoms and treatment. If you have questions about how the information in this book applies to your child, speak with your child's pediatrician.

Products mentioned in this book are for informational purposes only. Inclusion in this publication does not constitute or imply a guarantee or an endorsement by the American Academy of Pediatrics.

The information and advice in this book apply equally to children of both sexes (except where noted). To indicate this, we have chosen to alternate between masculine and feminine pronouns throughout the book.

Foreword

The American Academy of Pediatrics (AAP) welcomes you to the second edition of its popular parenting book, *Allergies and Asthma: What Every Parent Needs to Know.*

Although allergies and asthma can develop at any age, they most commonly show up during childhood or early adulthood. These conditions are explored in detail in *Allergies and Asthma: What Every Parent Needs to Know.* This book will help parents identify and avoid allergen and asthma triggers, prevent asthma attacks in their children, evaluate traditional and complementary forms of treatment and therapy, and understand how to alleviate and prevent symptoms.

What separates this book from other references on allergies and asthma is that pediatricians who specialize in these conditions have extensively reviewed it. Under the direction of our editor in chief, the material in this book was developed with the assistance of numerous reviewers and contributors from the AAP and its committees and sections. Because medical information is constantly changing, every effort has been made to ensure that this book contains the most up-to-date findings. Readers may want to visit the AAP Web site for parents, HealthyChildren.org, to keep current on this and other subjects.

It is the hope of the AAP that this book will become an invaluable resource and reference guide to parents. We are confident that parents and caregivers will find the book extremely valuable. We encourage its use along with the advice and counsel of our readers' pediatricians, who will provide individual guidance and assistance related to the health of children.

The AAP is an organization of 60,000 primary care pediatricians, pediatric medical subspecialists, and pediatric surgical specialists dedicated to the health, safety, and well-being of infants, children, adolescents, and young adults. *Allergies and Asthma: What Every Parent Needs to Know* is part of ongoing AAP educational efforts to provide parents and caregivers with high-quality information on a broad spectrum of children's health issues.

Errol R. Alden, MD, FAAP
Executive Director/CEO
American Academy of Pediatrics

PART 1
THE BASICS

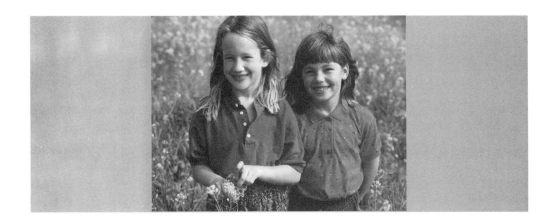

Chapter 1

Allergies and Asthma Explained

Allergies, eczema, and asthma often start in childhood and persist throughout life. Although none can be cured, with understanding and proper care they can usually be kept under control. While asthma and eczema are not primarily allergic diseases, allergies often play an important role in these 2 conditions.

Every fall, 5-year-old Timmy develops a runny nose; itchy, puffy eyes; and attacks of sneezing. His mother shares the problem, which she dismisses as mild hay fever and something her son has to learn to live with. Lately, however, Timmy has also suffered attacks of wheezing and shortness of breath when he visits his grandmother and plays with her cats. Timmy's pediatrician suspects allergic asthma and wants him to undergo some tests.

At first, Maria thought her baby daughter had heat rash. But the dry, itchy patches didn't go away, and even though Maria put mittens on little Jenine's hands, she couldn't prevent the baby from rubbing and scratching the rash areas until they were raw and infected.

When 6-year-old Tanisha developed red, itchy eyes, her mother assumed she had caught pinkeye (an eye infection) from a school friend. Her pediatrician prescribed antibiotic eyedrops, but 2 weeks later, Tanisha's eyes were as red and itchy as ever, leading her pediatrician to suspect allergies rather than an infection.

At age 15, Joshua collapsed after being stung by a bee while on a Boy Scouts camping trip. Fortunately, after a previous severe allergic reaction to a bee sting, Joshua's allergy specialist had prescribed an epinephrine (adrenaline) autoinjector. Joshua followed the doctor's instructions and kept it with him at all times in case of such an emergency. Realizing he was having an attack of anaphylaxis, Joshua was able to get out the autoinjector and give himself a lifesaving shot of epinephrine.

Then there's 7-year-old Jamie, who breaks out in itchy hives after eating peanuts. And 12-year-old Alex, who coughs and becomes really short of breath whenever he mows the lawn and has to run a mile in his gym class.

*A*lthough these brief case histories, collected from actual medical records, describe very different symptoms and situations, they have a common thread—all are related to allergies, which doctors sometimes call *atopic diseases* or *hypersensitivity reactions*. Indeed, allergies and asthma, which typically start in childhood, are by far the most common chronic diseases among children in the United States. Consider the following statistics:

- Some 50 million Americans have allergies (about 1 in 5 people in this country).
- The most common type of allergy is hay fever (allergic rhinitis); the medical cost of treating it, when direct and indirect costs are added up, now exceeds $7 billion a year.
- More than 17 million Americans have asthma, and about one-fourth of these are younger than 18 years. Asthma accounts for about 4,000 deaths a year.
- Seventy to 80% of school-aged children with asthma also have allergies, which are among the most common triggers for asthma, closely tied with viral respiratory infections.
- If one parent has allergies, there's a 25% chance that a child will also be allergic. The risk is more than doubled to 60% to 70% if both parents have allergies.

Many aspects of allergies, eczema, and asthma still are not fully understood. But advances in the diagnosis and treatment of these disorders are helping millions of sufferers. These will be discussed in the following chapters. But first, here's a brief overview of these all-too-common chronic disorders.

What Are Allergies?

Many people mistakenly use the word *allergy* to refer to a disease or almost any unpleasant or adverse reaction. We often hear someone say, "I have allergies," "He's allergic to hard work," or "She's allergic to anything that's green." In reality, allergies are reactions that are usually caused by an overactive immune system. These reactions can occur in a variety of organs in the body, resulting in diseases such as asthma, hay fever, and eczema.

Your immune system is made up of a number of different cells that come from organs throughout the body—principally bone marrow, the thymus gland, and a network of lymph nodes and lymph tissue scattered throughout the body, including the spleen, gastrointestinal tract, tonsils, and the adenoid (an olive-shaped structure that is located at the top of the throat behind the nose).

Normally, it's the immune system that protects the body against disease by searching out and destroying foreign invaders, such as viruses and bacteria. In an allergic reaction, the immune system overreacts and goes into action against a normally harmless substance, such as pollen or animal dander. These allergy-provoking substances are called *allergens*.

Bone marrow serves as a factory and storage house for white blood cells (leukocytes), as well as other types of blood cells. Some types of immature white blood cells, called *stem cells*, are carried to other parts of the immune system, where they develop into more specialized, disease-fighting cells. For example, T lymphocytes, or simply T cells, complete their development in the thymus, an organ located behind the breastbone that is made up of lymphoid

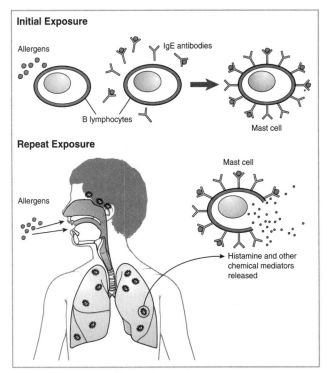

Initial Exposure

Allergens

IgE antibodies

B lymphocytes

Mast cell

Repeat Exposure

Mast cell

Allergens

Histamine and other chemical mediators released

On encountering an allergen for the first time, the body responds with B lymphocytes that secrete IgE antibodies against the allergen. These IgE antibodies then reside on the surface of mast cells, special cells found in everybody's skin, lung, nose, eye, and intestine lining that are filled with chemical mediators (potent molecules that "mediate" inflammation), known to be important in allergic inflammation. When the allergen comes into the body again (eg, in the nose, bronchial tubes, gastrointestinal tract), it binds to the IgE on mast cells, causing a release of the mast cells' potent chemicals, leading to local tissues becoming inflamed. This inflammation and other actions resulting from the mediators are what cause the various problems and symptoms seen in asthma, hay fever, anaphylaxis, food allergy, insect sting allergy, and medication (eg, antibiotic) allergy.

What Happens During an Allergic Reaction

1. The allergen enters the body; it may be inhaled (eg, pollen, dust mite, animal dander, mold), be swallowed (eg, certain food substances, penicillin and other medications), be injected (eg, bee venom, penicillin), or come into direct contact with the skin or eyes.

2. The immune system recognizes the substance as foreign and responds by producing an antibody called IgE. This antibody molecule is programmed to remember and act against the specific allergen.

3. The IgE molecules latch on to the surfaces of mast cells, a type of cell that usually serves to help promote inflammation to fight off infection. Mast cells are abundant in the connective tissue of the skin, upper airways and lungs, and lining of the stomach and intestines. A person will not experience an allergic reaction to this initial exposure, but if that person is vulnerable to allergies, the antibodies will stay on the alert for future encounters with the allergen.

4. If, at some future time, the allergen again enters the body, it links up with the IgE molecules on the mast cells.

5. When the allergen binds to the IgE molecule, a reaction occurs whereby tiny granules inside the mast cells are released. These granules contain very active substances (histamine and various other molecules) that cause the inflammation, swelling, itching, and other symptoms of an allergic response.

tissue. Mature T cells attack invading microorganisms directly and assist B lymphocytes, or B cells, in some of their effects.

B cells develop in the lymph nodes and other lymphatic tissue. These cells produce *antibodies*—highly specialized proteins that are programmed to recognize a specific foreign invader and go into action to destroy it whenever it enters the body. These antibodies are useful and beneficial to the body.

In a person with allergies, the immune system produces the usual and normal beneficial antibodies, but additional ones are made and directed against allergens; these antibodies interact with allergens and actually lead to the various allergic problems that plague children and adults. Here is a simplified overview of what happens in a typical allergic response.

Because mast cells are concentrated in the airways (eg, nose, throat, bronchial tubes), lining of the gastrointestinal tract, and skin, allergic reactions have their greatest effects on these parts of the body. Allergic responses vary greatly depending on the part of the body that is involved, and differ from one person to another and even within one person over time. Some people just suffer from hay fever (more correctly termed *allergic rhinitis),* others from *allergic* asthma, and yet others have combinations of different allergy manifestations or conditions (see "Symptoms Associated With Allergies" on the next page). The reason for this variety of symptoms (manifestations) is unknown. It is important to realize that rhinitis and asthma can occur without evidence of allergy (ie, due to other nonallergic causes).

Sometimes it takes years of exposure to an allergen before symptoms appear. Take, for example, the case of Reggie. Over the years, he had been given penicillin several times for childhood infections. When he was in college, he developed a severe strep throat and was given a course of penicillin to take by mouth. Within minutes of the first dose, Reggie developed extensive hives (itchy welts). Antihistamines calmed this allergic reaction, and Reggie was warned that in the future he should wear a medical identification tag to let health care workers know that he is allergic to penicillin. Further use of the medication might result in an even more severe reaction called *anaphylaxis,* which can be fatal (see "Warning" on the next page).

This, of course, is an extreme example. Most allergies can be kept in check by a combination of identifying and avoiding potential allergens, together with the use of various medications.

Who Is at Risk?

Although allergies can develop at any age, they most commonly show up during childhood or early adulthood. A search of family medical histories of a child with allergies will usually turn up a close relative who also has allergies. If one parent, brother, or sister has allergies, there is a 25% chance that a child will also have allergies. The risk is much higher if both parents are allergic. But the child will not necessarily be allergic to the same substances as the parents or always show the same type of allergic disease (eg, hay fever, asthma, eczema).

Warning

Anaphylaxis—a rare but by far the most severe allergic reaction—is a life-threatening medical emergency that requires immediate treatment to prevent death. Symptoms usually occur immediately (within minutes) after exposure. Signs and symptoms include widespread swelling; difficulty breathing because of swelling of the mouth, throat, or bronchial tubes; wheezing; racing or pounding heart; cramping; diarrhea; agitation and anxiety; and loss of consciousness. For a more detailed discussion of anaphylaxis, see Chapter 6.

Symptoms Associated With Allergies

Eyes, Ears, Nose, Mouth
- Red, teary, or itchy eyes
- Puffiness around the eyes
- Sneezing
- Runny nose
- Itchy nose, nose rubbing
- Postnasal drip
- Nasal swelling and congestion
- Itchy ear canals
- Itching of the mouth and throat

Lungs
- Hacking dry cough or cough that produces clear mucus
- Wheezing (noisy breathing)
- Feeling of tightness in the chest
- Low exercise tolerance
- Rapid breathing; shortness of breath

Skin
- Eczema (patches of itchy, red skin rash)
- Hives (welts)

Intestines
- Cramps and intestinal discomfort
- Diarrhea
- Nausea or vomiting

Miscellaneous
- Headache
- Feelings of restlessness, irritability
- Excessive fatigue

When to Suspect an Allergy

As demonstrated in the examples at the beginning of this chapter, allergies can result in various types of conditions. Some are easy to identify by the pattern of symptoms that invariably follows exposure to a particular substance; others are more subtle and may masquerade as other conditions. Here are some common clues that should lead you to suspect your child may have an allergy.

- Patches of bumps or itchy, red skin that won't go away (see Chapter 3)
- Development of *hives*—intensely itchy skin eruptions that usually last for a few hours and move from one part of the body to another (see chapters 3 and 5)
- Repeated or chronic cold-like symptoms, such as a runny nose, nasal stuffiness, sneezing, and throat clearing, that last more than a week or two, or develop at about the same time every year (see Chapter 4)
- Nose rubbing, sniffling, snorting, sneezing, or drippy nose (see Chapter 4)
- Itchy, runny eyes (see Chapter 4)
- Itching or tingling sensations in the mouth and throat (see Chapter 5)
- Coughing, wheezing, difficulty breathing, and other respiratory symptoms (see Chapter 8)
- Unexplained bouts of diarrhea, abdominal cramps, and other intestinal symptoms (see Chapter 5)

Where Does Asthma Fit In?

Although allergies can trigger asthma and asthma is often associated with allergies, they are actually 2 different things. In simple terms, asthma is a chronic condition originating in the lungs, whereas allergies describe reactions that originate in the immune system and can affect many organs, including the lungs. Many different substances and circumstances can trigger an asthma attack—exercise, exposure to cold air, a viral infection, air pollution, noxious fumes, tobacco smoke, and for many asthma sufferers, a host of allergens. In fact, about 80% of children with asthma also have allergies. Although allergies are important in triggering asthma, severe asthma exacerbations are often set off by the good old common cold virus, totally unrelated to allergy. Here are a few real-life examples of how asthma can appear.

Ed and his wife, Mary Alice, suffer from allergic reactions—Ed is very allergic to cats, ragweed pollen, and dust mites, causing ongoing nasal congestion and runny nose, while hay fever makes spring a misery for Mary Alice. At first, they thought that their son Danny had escaped his parents' allergies. He didn't have a trace of eczema or unusual sneezing, sniffling, or other allergy symptoms, even when he played with a neighbor's cat. At about age 3, however, Danny developed a persistent cough that seemed to worsen at night. Then Danny caught a bad cold, and just when he seemed to be recovering nicely, he began wheezing and breathing with great difficulty. Mary Alice immediately called her pediatrician, who told her to bring Danny to the emergency department. Doctors there quickly determined that Danny was having an attack of asthma. Prompt treatment brought the episode under control, but that flare-up marked the beginning of a long struggle to keep Danny's asthma in check.

Michelle's story is quite different. Neither of her parents has allergies and there is no family history of asthma on either side. When Michelle was about 2 years old, her parents noticed that she wheezed and coughed a lot, sometimes triggered by colds, but not always. They thought the problem was simply a prolonged "cold" and so were shocked when their pediatrician told them Michelle had asthma.

Nine-year-old Rodney, a budding soccer player, seemed to live for the sport. But his junior league coach was concerned about the shortness of breath that often forced a very frustrated Rodney to take to the sidelines. The coach urged Rodney's parents to consult their pediatrician, who diagnosed the young athlete's problem as exercise-induced asthma.

These brief case histories illustrate just a few of the many ways in which asthma can manifest itself. But regardless of the manner of onset, what happens in the lungs is pretty much the same. The *bronchi*—the tubes that carry air in and out of the lungs—are abnormally hypersensitive. It turns out that everybody's bronchi are capable of becoming narrow, or constricted, possibly to protect the lungs against the entry of harmful substances. In asthma, the bronchi are overly sensitive and tighten up in the presence of normally harmless substances. Many doctors describe asthmatic bronchi as "twitchy."

But there's another side to asthma. The hypersensitive bronchi become inflamed, which results in internal swelling and increased production of mucus. This inflammation, in turn, is important in making the bronchi twitchy. When bronchi develop low-grade, long-standing inflammation, the result is chronic asthma. Tightening of the bronchi, along with inflammation and swelling, makes it doubly difficult to breathe. The child with this condition may complain of a tight feeling in the chest, have a deep cough, or develop wheezing (a whistling noise) from the lungs.

Use of an inhaled *bronchodilator*—medication that relaxes the muscles controlling the bronchi—can usually eliminate asthma symptoms quickly when they occur. Other medications are given to stop the ongoing inflammation. Very often, medications are used daily, even when the asthma seems to be quiet, to calm the twitchy bronchi and control inflammation. The proper use of asthma medications, coupled with lifestyle changes that come from identifying and avoiding as many allergen and other asthma triggers as possible, is the key to successful asthma control. For a more detailed discussion of all aspects of asthma, see chapters 8 through 13.

Chapter 2

Determining the Problem

*O*ne *common pattern of allergy-related problems starts in infancy with eczema and food allergy. Next follows a phase often marked by recurrent infections of the ears, throat, and sinuses with upper respiratory symptoms. Finally, obvious—or not so obvious—symptoms of hay fever or asthma may appear.*

Seven-year-old Johnny has been diagnosed with recurrent bronchitis since he was only a few months old. In a typical episode, Johnny starts coughing, then wheezing, and finally, his chest becomes congested and he has trouble breathing. At the clinic where his family receives medical care, the doctors routinely prescribe an antibiotic to clear up the bacterial infection they believe is causing the bronchitis. Johnny also gets an inhaler medication to relieve the cough and make it easier to breathe. Johnny asks his mother for a dose of this "cough medicine" almost every day.

Johnny's bronchitis attacks have become more frequent and severe in the 3 years since he started school. His mother also notices that Johnny starts wheezing whenever he runs or plays hard. Johnny often misses school because of his chest problems and bronchitis.

In addition to Johnny's coughing and wheezing, he has a nonstop runny nose, his eyes and nose are itchy, and he complains that his ears are blocked. At Johnny's last clinic visit, the doctor sent him for radiographs, which showed that he had *sinusitis,* an inflammation of the sinuses (air spaces in the bones of the face that connect with the nasal passages). This condition is often but not always caused by a bacterial infection. After yet another course of antibiotic treatment, his symptoms improved a little but did not completely go away.

For years, Johnny's mother has told herself that the youngster will grow out of his symptoms, but instead they are getting worse. On learning that both parents have hay fever and that Johnny's mother has asthma, the clinic doctor asks Johnny's mother to make a special follow-up visit to discuss the possibility that Johnny has asthma and allergies. After this visit, the pediatrician decides to refer him to a pediatric allergy specialist for testing and a medical opinion.

· ·

First, the History

Diagnosis follows an orderly process that starts with a careful medical history. Your pediatrician or allergy specialist will ask a lot of questions about your child's symptoms and medical background, and about your family's medical history as well.

- Does your child cough, wheeze, or get extra short of breath when she's running or playing hard?
- Does your child cough a lot? Is the coughing worse at night? Is she wheezing? Does she have trouble breathing? Does her chest feel tight sometimes?
- What happens when she laughs or becomes upset?
- Does your child sneeze frequently? Does she rub her nose often? Does she blow her nose or wipe it a lot? Is the nasal discharge clear and runny? (A clear discharge is typical of allergic rhinitis, also called hay fever, the most common form of allergy; see "Allergic Rhinitis and Asthma" on page 34.) Or is it thick and greenish or yellowish? (A yellow or green color suggests that your child may have an infection, separate or possibly in addition to allergy symptoms.)

Symptoms: All in the Timing

Allergy symptoms that come and go with the seasons may be caused by seasonal plants such as trees, grasses, and weeds. Coughing, sneezing, or other chest and nose symptoms that get much better when your child is away from home may indicate that your child is sensitive to substances normally found indoors, such as pets. By contrast, symptoms that always clear up on weekends and school vacations suggest that there may be a problem with something in the environment at school.

Coughing at night with hoarseness and frequent throat clearing may be caused by postnasal drip from allergic rhinitis or sinusitis. But coughing, wheezing, and related symptoms that get worse at night may also raise suspicions about asthma because asthma symptoms are often worse at night. Your pediatrician may suspect exercise-induced asthma if your child frequently coughs or wheezes when running or playing energetically.

- Are her eyes itchy and watery?
- Does she have more than her share of colds? Do they last longer than a week?
- Does she ever have a rash or itchy bumps on the skin?
- How often does she have symptoms? How long do they last?
- Do particular events or exposures seem to bring on symptoms, or make them better or worse? (See "Symptoms: All in the Timing" above.)
- Have the symptoms ever gotten better after your child has taken medicine? What kind of medication helped?

Your pediatrician will ask whether your child's symptoms often appear during a particular season of the year, at a certain location, or when your child is around animals, such as cats. Your pediatrician will also ask whether symptoms come on after your child has eaten a particular food.

Your pediatrician will ask whether other members of the family have hay fever, asthma, or eczema because allergy and asthma run in families (see "Allergies Tend to Run in Families" below). However, even if you can't recall a single relative who sneezes and wheezes, your doctor will not discount allergy and asthma in your child because, like many disorders, they can appear with no prior family history.

Parents sometimes try over-the-counter medications before asking their pediatricians about a persistent cough, a rash, or respiratory symptoms. Although it's recommended that you talk with your pediatrician before giving medications to your child, it's helpful to tell the doctor whether a medication had any effect because this can give clues about the possible cause of symptoms. For example, if a runny nose and itchiness bothered your child less and she stopped sneezing for a while after taking an antihistamine, chances are she has an allergy and not an infection. Conversely, if her coughing and wheezing did not change after she took a dose of an over-the-counter medication, your pediatrician may decide to test or even go ahead and treat for asthma before looking for other underlying conditions.

Allergies Tend to Run in Families

Many types of allergy problems, including hay fever, asthma, and eczema, tend to run in families. If both parents have allergies, each child has about a 60% to 70% chance of being allergic.

However, allergic responses to insect venom, medications, and latex are the exceptions to the rule. Having a parent with one of these allergies does not increase the chance a child will be allergic.

Then, the Physical Examination

Your child's weight and height will be measured and compared with his records to make sure he is growing and gaining weight at a satisfactory rate. Your pediatrician will note whether your child is breathing through the mouth because of a stuffed-up nose. The doctor will also look for *allergic shiners*—bruise-like discolorations below the eyes that are frequently signs of chronic nasal blockage. Another reason may simply be that the same allergies creating a nose problem can result in inflammation in the eyes, leading to the discoloration. These signs may indicate that your child has allergic rhinitis or allergic conjunctivitis, often referred to as hay fever (see Chapter 4).

A child whose nose is always running may unconsciously make a gesture that has been termed the *allergic salute*—a quick upward swipe to the nose. By pushing the nose upward dozens of times a day, some children actually develop a permanent crease (commonly called an *allergic crease)* across the nose where the pliable cartilage meets the bony bridge. Your pediatrician will look inside your child's nose to see if the lining is swollen and pale, a finding typical of allergies. Your pediatrician will also note the color of the mucus because discharge caused by allergies is normally clear or white.

Your doctor will look for redness caused by allergic inflammation in the whites of your child's eyes and for bumps on the lining of the eyelids, which can be signs of allergies. Examination of the chest may show an unusual barrel shape, which is sometimes a sign of asthma. Using the stethoscope, your doctor will listen for wheezes and other unusual sounds that may be heard in asthma. Your pediatrician will look over your child's skin for rashes, particularly dry, scratched-over patches near the joints, which can indicate eczema.

Finally, the Tests

Blood Tests
Blood tests may be ordered—first, for an indication of your child's general health, and second, to count the numbers of *eosinophils,* a type of white blood cell involved in allergic responses. An unusually high eosinophil count points to possible allergies.

Your pediatrician may also order a total allergy antibody test, called an *IgE level* (see Chapter 1, page 5). The total IgE level does not detect specific allergies. However, if the total IgE level is higher than normal, there's a strong possibility that your child has allergies. However, a normal total IgE level does not necessarily mean you do not have allergies; it is only helpful when it is elevated. Skin testing or a blood test (see "Specific IgE Blood Test [RAST]" on page 16) needs to be done to specifically identify what triggers the allergies. Your pediatrician may refer you to a pediatric allergist for these tests.

Skin Tests
Skin tests, first developed almost a century ago, are still the mainstay of allergy testing. They are easy and safe to do, give fast results, and are relatively inexpensive, which makes them the best way to start looking for specific allergies.

In performing *scratch* skin tests, drops of allergen extracts (eg, pollens, dust mites, molds, animal danders, foods) are allowed to seep through shallow scratches made in the patient's skin. The tests can also be performed by the deeper, *intradermal* technique, in which extracts are injected under the skin. There are pros and cons to both testing methods. Scratch tests are painless and very easy to do. They are somewhat less sensitive than intradermal tests; they are also less likely to cause a severe reaction in someone who is highly allergic. The intradermal tests, which let the allergen extracts penetrate deeper into the skin, are highly sensitive, but they can occasionally result in false-positive reactions, indicating allergies where none exist. Your physician may decide to start with scratch tests, then go on to intradermal testing if further information is needed. Before testing, your doctor will ask you not to give your child any antihistamines for 3 to 5 days, as they will interfere with the results of the tests.

Skin Tests Must Be Done by an Experienced Physician

Although a positive result to scratch or intradermal skin testing strongly suggests that your child has formed IgE antibodies against a specific allergen, it does not follow that your child will definitely develop allergy symptoms when exposed to that particular allergen in the environment. As a rule, the bigger the skin test reaction, the higher the chances are that your child is allergic and will sneeze, itch, or break out in a rash. However, in some cases the skin reaction is trivial while the symptoms are overwhelming, and vice versa. Further, even though your child may have diminished symptoms as he gets older, the skin test result can remain positive. It is important that tests be conducted and results interpreted by someone trained and experienced in allergy skin testing.

If your child has formed specific IgE antibodies through earlier exposure to one of the substances being tested, the skin test area will redden and swell into a disk that looks like a mosquito bite around the puncture site. This skin reaction usually peaks within 15 to 20 minutes after the test extracts are applied, and then gradually clears up. The skin where the tests were done may feel itchy for a few hours.

This Is Only a Test

Many parents and children are afraid of having allergy skin testing because they've heard false reports that it is painful and upsetting. Scratch tests, the form of testing most often used in children, are mostly painless because they are done on the surface of the skin, where there aren't any nerve endings to register pain. Furthermore, new test devices are available that can do up to 8 tests at a time and allow scratch testing to be done quickly and without injury. The intradermal technique uses a very fine needle to penetrate the surface of the skin. It is "felt" a little more than scratch testing but is still not very painful.

Many people also falsely believe that children have to reach a certain age before they can be tested. In fact, age is no barrier to skin testing; positive results can be obtained at any age. For example, in infants and toddlers who have eczema and suspected food allergy, skin tests often reveal sensitivity to milk or egg. Once parents have this information, they can keep those foods out of their child's diet to control allergy symptoms.

Finally, experienced doctors and nurses perform allergy testing on a daily basis. They know how to take away fears and put children—and parents—at ease.

Specific IgE Blood Test (RAST)

Instead of skin tests, your pediatrician or allergy specialist may order a blood test that has various names, including specific IgE blood test, in vitro IgE test, and radioallergosorbent test (RAST). (When the test was first invented years ago, it was called RAST, based on the specific way the test was done in the laboratory. Even though that technique is no longer used, the name RAST has kind of hung on.) The specific IgE blood test is especially useful if skin tests cannot be done because, for instance, a child has eczema over much of his body or cannot be taken off medication that interferes with skin testing. This blood test shows specific sensitivities, as skin tests do, but does so by detecting the presence of allergy antibodies circulating in the blood. If antibodies are in the blood, it usually means the same antibodies are also in other tissues. The method is not quite as versatile as skin testing because certain extracts are not available for measuring specific IgE using this technique. For example, a specific IgE blood test cannot be used to detect sensitivity to medications and is rarely used to detect insect venom allergy. However, the specific IgE blood test, in general, is adaptable and sensitive enough to detect a wide range of allergies.

The procedure costs more per test than skin testing. It requires only a few minutes of the patient's time to draw a blood sample and there is no risk of any allergic reaction. The results take from 1 to 5 days, whereas skin test results are available immediately.

Radiographs and Imaging Tests

While sometimes useful, radiographs (x-ray films) are not essential for diagnosing asthma or allergies. In fact, people with asthma usually have normal chest radiographs. However, chest radiographs are sometimes done to make sure children do not have other conditions that can mimic asthma.

Sinus infection can produce symptoms similar to those of respiratory allergies, and children who have respiratory allergies are prone to sinus infections. Your pediatrician may order an imaging test to see if your child simply has a prolonged or recurrent infection, or whether a sinus infection is complicating his allergies. An imaging test can be done the old-fashioned way, with a radiograph of the head, or it can be performed by computed tomography (CT). A CT scan is more sensitive than a radiograph and shows finer details of the anatomy of the sinuses, which can help your pediatrician decide on the best way to treat your child's sinus problem.

Finally, imaging tests can sometimes help your pediatrician identify the reason your child snores or has a permanently stuffed-up nose. A radiograph of the upper neck area can show if the stuffiness is caused by enlargement of the adenoid tissue, which sits in the upper throat just behind the nose.

Lung Function Tests

If your child has symptoms indicating possible asthma, your pediatrician or asthma specialist may perform tests to evaluate his lung function. Lung function tests are performed in your pediatrician's office or a pulmonary function laboratory where special equipment is available. An instrument called a *spirometer* is used to measure how much air your child can breathe out, as well as how fast the air flows. The technician will place a clip over your child's nose to prevent air escaping from the nostrils. The technician will then ask your child to perform breathing maneuvers into a mouthpiece attached to a pulmonary function monitor. The maneuvers aren't difficult or painful. All your child has to do is take a deep breath, then breathe out forcefully through the mouthpiece. Instead of using a spirometer, the doctor may ask your child to blow into a simpler device called a *peak flow meter* (see Chapter 11, page 108). Your pediatrician usually has your child perform the lung function test at least 3 times at a sitting to make sure results are consistent.

Asthma Screening

The American College of Allergy, Asthma & Immunology conducts an annual Nationwide Asthma Screening Program for children and adults in more than 200 communities. Allergists, who are asthma specialists, will conduct the free screenings, which take place in May (National Asthma and Allergy Awareness Month). To find out where screening is available, visit www.acaai.org and click on "Patient Educational Resources" in the "Patients & Public" menu, or write Asthma Screening Program, ACAAI, 85 W Alonquin Rd, Suite 550, Arlington Heights, IL 60005.

If lung function testing shows that your child cannot blow air out fast enough, your pediatrician may perform further tests for asthma. Your pediatrician may give your child a dose of bronchodilator medication to see if there is a change in airflow. If airflow is normal or improved after the medication, the result strongly suggests that asthma is present.

Food Diary

If your pediatrician suspects that your child has a food allergy, you may be asked to keep a food diary for several weeks. Use the diary to write down every single food your child eats and any symptoms that follow within minutes to a few hours after a particular meal or snack.

The food diary may be used together with an elimination diet. Your pediatrician will give you a list of foods to keep out of your child's diet for a certain period. You may then be instructed to reintroduce each food one at a time at intervals of several days, using the diary to note any symptoms that recur or appear for the first time. This method, called *food avoidance and rechallenge,* may help to establish whether a specific food allergy is present.

If your pediatrician has any concerns about the possibility of a life-threatening anaphylactic reaction to a food (see Chapter 6), you will be instructed not to reintroduce the suspect food at home. Instead, your pediatrician or pediatric allergist may perform a food challenge test, if required, in the clinic setting where emergency care is available. However, if your child's history is highly suspicious, such a challenge may be too dangerous and will not be done at all.

A food challenge is sometimes done to double-check the results of skin testing or a specific IgE blood test (especially when results are negative), or when the food avoidance and rechallenge method has not provided enough information. Under close observation in the allergy specialist's office, your child will be asked to swallow small but increasing amounts of the suspect food. Allergy symptoms, which typically appear anywhere from 5 to 60 minutes after eating the food, are looked for. If there is no reaction even after eating the largest amount of food given in the challenge, it is concluded the child has outgrown the allergy to that food.

Sweat Test

Cystic fibrosis is an inherited disorder that involves many body systems. It causes symptoms in the respiratory and digestive tracts that can mimic those of asthma and allergies. A child with cystic fibrosis may have asthma or allergies, as well. Your pediatrician may order tests to measure the levels of certain minerals in your child's sweat (commonly called a *sweat test*). If the results indicate cystic fibrosis, further tests will be done to confirm the diagnosis.

What Happens Next?

After making an initial diagnosis of allergy on the basis of the history and symptoms, and performing skin tests or a blood allergy test, your child's pediatrician or allergy specialist will advise on the best course of treatment. If your child's symptoms don't improve after a trial of treatment, further tests may be warranted.

PART 2
RECOGNIZING AND DEALING WITH ALLERGIES

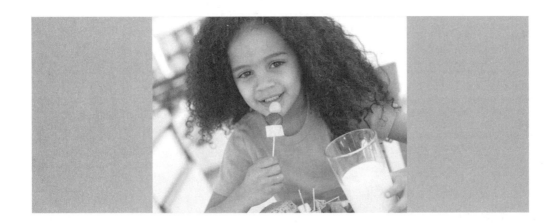

Chapter 3

Skin Allergies

*T*he most common chronic inflammatory skin condition in children is eczema, also
called atopic dermatitis. Although not strictly an allergic disorder, eczema in young children
has many of the hallmarks of allergies and is often a harbinger of hay fever and asthma. The
rate of eczema, like that of asthma, is increasing throughout the world. Hives, another common
rash in children, is clearly different from eczema and can represent an allergic reaction to a
food, an insect, or a medication trigger, but in many cases, no definite allergy cause is
ever found.

When Christine was 6 months old, her mother weaned her from breast milk to a cow's-milk–based formula. Christine had occasionally spat up, but now she started vomiting after being fed. At the same time, a dry, crusty rash appeared on her cheeks, then spread behind her ears, onto her neck, and over her arms and legs. Christine, normally a happy infant, seemed irritable with the rash. Her mother often found Christine rubbing her face against the sheets even while she slept, which made the rash worse. The vomiting stopped when Christine's pediatrician switched her to a low-allergenic formula made with hydrolyzed protein. He explained that Christine's rash was *atopic dermatitis,* commonly called eczema, often an early sign of allergy problems. The doctor prescribed a low-strength cortisone cream and a sedating antihistamine to be given at bedtime. Regular use of these medications helped keep the rash under control.

The rash became worse after Christine had her first fried egg, at around age 1. After this, her parents were careful to keep eggs out of her diet, but occasionally a dish made with a small amount of egg, such as noodles, slipped past them. Christine's eczema always flared up right after she ate a food containing egg.

By Christine's third birthday, her skin rash was gradually getting better, but her mother called the pediatrician when Christine started wheezing during a cold, as the doctor had warned she might. Even after her cold cleared up, Christine had frequent chest rattles and cough, and a constant stuffy nose.

Eczema: Not Quite Allergy?

Eczema has some puzzling features that don't fit neatly into the pattern we recognize as allergy. For example, children with eczema usually have high blood levels of IgE, the antibody involved in allergic reactions. However, their allergy skin tests don't always reveal evidence of allergy, or if they do, the substances in question are not always important factors in the eczema.

By the time Christine was ready for kindergarten at age 5, her eczema was completely gone. However, her pediatrician had diagnosed chronic asthma and hay fever. These conditions were kept under control with regular use of medications.

*F*or many parents, the first sign in allergies of all kinds that they should be on the watch for is a single patch of fine bumps or a dry, red, crusty rash that starts on their baby's cheeks and spreads over most of the face and body. The "look" of eczema varies—although it can appear weepy, it is more commonly dry, scaly, or crusty. The rash is intensely itchy— a hallmark of eczema. In fact, itching can sometimes set in before a rash appears. The discomfort may change the baby's mood; an infant or toddler who was formerly content may become continually irritable.

Eczema affects between 5% and 10% of children and usually—but not always—disappears before adulthood. However, in many cases, as children outgrow eczema they develop typical symptoms of respiratory allergy, such as hay fever (see Chapter 4) or asthma (see chapters 8–13). About 50% to 75% of children with eczema develop another form or type of allergy problem at some point. Children tend to develop asthma at an earlier age if they start out with eczema. Interestingly, though, about 20% of all patients with eczema never have any sign of allergies and they usually do not have a family history of allergy problems.

Psoriasis: Not Eczema, Not Allergy

A school-aged child may develop an itchy rash that spreads and joins up to form irregular patches, most often on the elbows, knees, and scalp, or around the navel. Eventually, the patches become covered with thick white scales.

These patches are typical of *psoriasis*. Unlike eczema, psoriasis is not an allergic condition. Frequently, there is a family history of psoriasis, and the child may have had unusually extensive cradle cap in infancy or dandruff in the toddler and preschool years. The condition occurs in both sexes but is more common in girls. Attacks of psoriasis are often linked to periods of emotional stress, such as examination time at school. In some children, psoriasis may follow strep throat.

Do not try to remove the scales or treat the condition with over-the-counter remedies. If your pediatrician diagnoses psoriasis, your child may be referred to a dermatologist.

Most children with eczema develop their skin symptoms in their first 1 to 2 years of life, and almost all before age 5 years. The pattern of symptoms differs according to children's ages. In infants and young children, the rash generally appears on the face (except around the nose), scalp, abdomen, arms, and legs. It may appear on the trunk and back but almost never spreads to the diaper area (see "Diaper Rash Is Not Eczema" on page 24). Before 4 to 6 months of age, infants don't have the muscular coordination to scratch the itch. Instead, they try to ease the intense discomfort by rubbing their faces against bedclothes or the sides of their cribs. This can break the skin surface, sometimes causing weeping and crusting, and the baby becomes even more uncomfortable, especially if the broken skin becomes infected. In older children, the eczema rash is usually confined to the neck and to the skin folds and large joints, such as the creases of the elbows and knees. In more severe cases, the rash affects the wrists, hands, ankles, and feet (but not the palms and soles).

Diaper Rash Is Not Eczema

If your baby has a crusty rash in the diaper area, consult your pediatrician. A diaper rash is rarely due to the child having eczema. Treatment may be required to soothe the irritation and clear up an infection. Protect against diaper rash with a zinc oxide cream. Avoid using commercial wet wipes, which may contain irritating compounds. Clean your baby with plain warm water.

Over time and with constant scratching, the eczematous skin can become dry, darker, and thickened, and the normal surface lines are deeper. These scarring-type changes are called *lichenification.*

A Crusty Rash May Be Impetigo

The rash of eczema can sometimes break, weep, and form a crusty scab. If these skin changes are significant and out of the ordinary, your child may have *impetigo.* This is a skin infection caused by *Streptococcus* or *Staphylococcus* bacteria. Call your pediatrician; if your child has impetigo, antibiotic treatment is required to clear up the condition and prevent it from spreading to others.

Identifying Triggers

Your pediatrician considers many factors in looking for the cause of eczema. Researchers estimate that food allergy plays a role in about 25% of cases of eczema in young children. The protein in egg white is the most common food allergy trigger after infancy. However, the atypical nature of eczema can make it difficult to pinpoint a specific food sensitivity. Allergy skin testing or a blood allergy test can sometimes be helpful. Alternatively, your pediatrician may simply review your child's history and suggest that you withhold a suspect food or try a low-allergenic diet for 10 to 14 days to see if symptoms improve. If you don't see a change for the better after this trial, foods probably don't play a role in your child's skin troubles. You should try these measures only on your pediatrician's advice to make sure that your child is getting the nutrients she needs. For example, if your pediatrician advises you to keep milk and dairy foods out of the diet, your pediatrician may recommend alternative sources of calcium and vitamins.

Although children with eczema may develop respiratory allergies later on, sensitivity to airborne allergens such as pollen and mold spores does not seem to be an important trigger for eczema. However, in a subset of children with eczema, the rash may be brought on or worsened by contact with dust mites and animal dander.

The rash of eczema can be aggravated by many nonallergenic environmental conditions, such as wide swings in temperature or humidity, extremely dry air, scratchy or tight clothing, and sweating. Many children with eczema cannot tolerate wool next to their skin. Skin symptoms, especially scratching, sometimes get worse when a youngster is overtired, nervous, or emotionally upset.

In getting to the source of your child's eczema, your pediatrician will look for other possible causes of an itchy, scaling rash. In young infants, cradle cap, or seborrheic dermatitis, can resemble eczema. However, cradle cap usually appears before 6 weeks of age and does not make the baby itchy and irritable. Parasites, such as lice and scabies, and irritating substances can produce similar symptoms, but the distribution of the rash is different from the characteristic pattern of eczema. These conditions usually clear up quite rapidly with treatment. Extremely severe eczema may be a sign that an infant has a severe underlying condition (such as an immune deficiency) that should be investigated.

Managing Eczema

In addition to the dietary approaches mentioned previously, your pediatrician can recommend measures to help clear up the rash and itching. Antihistamine medication may be prescribed to relieve the itching and help break the itch-scratch cycle (which leads to more itching, scratching, and possibly infection). Your pediatrician may advise giving the medication at night; some antihistamines have the side effect of mild drowsiness, which can help the child sleep better and suppress the urge to scratch during sleep. A non-sedating antihistamine can be used during the day when your child needs to stay alert for school. Long-sleeved sleepwear may also help to prevent nighttime scratching.

Choose Soaps and Detergents With Care

Soaps containing perfumes and deodorants may be too harsh for children's sensitive skin, especially children with eczema. Many pediatricians recommend non-soap cleansing lotions for infants and neutral, unscented, full-fat soaps or glycerin soaps for toddlers and older children. Children who cannot tolerate woolen clothing next to the skin may also be hypersensitive to lanolin-based soaps and lotions.

Use laundry products that are free of dyes and perfumes, and double-rinse clothes, towels, and bedding. If you have concerns about any personal care product, don't use it on your child.

A cortisone medication will be prescribed to reduce inflammation. This usually needs to be applied regularly (once or twice a day) to control the rash. Cortisone creams and ointments are available in various strengths. Some are too strong to be applied to the face and certain other parts of the body. These and all medications must be used exactly as prescribed to prevent side effects.

Warm (never hot) showers may be preferable to baths. In addition, moisturizing baths in lukewarm water for 20 minutes add moisture to the epithelial layer and cleanse the skin by lowering the number of bacteria. Gently pat your child dry after the shower or bath to allow some water to remain on the skin. Apply a moisturizer or lubricating cream to the whole body within 3 minutes, while the skin is still moist. This helps to keep the skin from drying out. Your child may also benefit from *wet wraps,* particularly if your child is an infant or a toddler (see "Wet-Wrap Therapy" on page 26).

Wet-Wrap Therapy

As the name implies, wet-wrap therapy involves wrapping wet bandages around the affected skin. This is generally done before bedtime.

The benefits of wet-wrap therapy include

- Skin rehydration
- More restful sleep
- Reduced redness and inflammation
- Less-frequent itching
- Decrease in the *Staphylococcus aureus* (staph) bacteria found on the skin

The basic technique is as follows:

1. The patient soaks in a bath with bath oil.
2. After bathing, pat the skin partially dry with a towel.
3. Apply moisturizer and eczema medication (eg, steroid crème, ointment) to rash areas.
4. Moisten bandages (eg, tubular bandage, wrap gauze bandage, athletic sock) by soaking them in water or applying moisturizer. When treating an infant or a very young child, moistened pajamas may be used instead of wet wraps. Special care must be taken to prevent these children from becoming chilled.
5. Wrap the wet bandages on the area to be treated. Wet bandages can be used on any area of the body that the patient will tolerate, including the face.
6. Lock in moisture by applying dry bandages over the wet ones.

The bandages should be left overnight but for no longer than 24 hours.

Clothing Shouldn't Get Under Your Child's Skin

Some synthetic fabrics, silk, and dyes and other chemicals used in manufacturing can irritate sensitive skin. Wash new clothes thoroughly before your child wears them. Look for T-shirts and underwear made of undyed cotton that your child can wear next to the skin. Cut off labels and turn undergarments inside out to keep scratchy seams and trimmings from irritating your child's skin. Use cotton sheets and blankets.

The more your child scratches, the greater the risk of the skin becoming infected. An antibiotic given by mouth or in the form of an ointment to rub on the skin may be necessary to clear up the infection. Antibiotic treatment may help to improve the rash as well, since the staphylococcus bacteria that commonly cause skin infections also trigger eczema in some cases. Keep your child's fingernails clean and short to reduce the risk of injury from scratching and prevent contamination of open scratches. Call your pediatrician promptly if your child's rash gets worse or recurs despite treatment.

Hives

Jeremy, 4 years old, has a bad cold and a bronchial infection, which keep him awake with coughing through the night. His pediatrician prescribes amoxicillin, an antibiotic, to clear up the bronchial infection. Five days after the start of the cold, Jeremy breaks out in hives. His body is covered in the typical rash of large and small itchy welts. Believing that the hives are an allergic reaction to the antibiotic, the doctor stops the medication and prescribes a different antibiotic as well as an antihistamine to stop the itching and swelling, and the hives gradually disappear.

Jeremy has no problems until 6 months later, when he catches another cold and again develops hives. This time he's not taking an antibiotic. Antihistamine treatment helps, but the hives take about 2 weeks to disappear completely. During each bout of hives, the welts are especially numerous around Jeremy's waist and the tops of his thighs, where the elastic in his underwear presses on the skin. The results of allergy testing do not indicate sensitivity to amoxicillin or the related antibiotic, penicillin, which are common causes of allergy. And according to the tests, Jeremy does not have any other allergies. After these early episodes, Jeremy never has another bout of hives.

$\mathcal{A}$t least 1 child in 5 has a bout of the itchy welts known as *hives,* or urticaria, at one time or another. Hives are intensely itchy, raised welts that resemble mosquito bites or the rash caused by stinging nettles. The welts usually appear in clusters and may run together to form a single large, raised swelling. Whether isolated or joined up, individual welts usually disappear anywhere from 2 to 24 hours after first emerging. However, new hives promptly appear on another part of the body to begin the cycle over again.

Often, hives are accompanied by *angioedema,* a deeper, more diffuse swelling that comes and goes with the same baffling unpredictability as the itchy welts. Hives appear most often on the trunk and limbs but may pop up anywhere. In contrast, angioedema usually affects loose tissue, such as the cheeks, lips, tongue, and skin around the eyes, although it can appear on the limbs as well. Angioedema is not usually itchy but may feel painful, burning, or simply strange. The swellings of angioedema come and go, as hives do, and may occur whether hives are present or not.

Although there may well be a specific cause for the hives or angioedema, it's not always possible to identify it before the rash burns itself out. Therefore, if your child has an isolated bout, your pediatrician will concentrate on relieving the annoying symptoms, rather than lose time in looking for the cause. However, if hives recur or become chronic—that is, an episode lasts longer than 6 weeks—it is worthwhile to look for the trigger factors so that preventive measures can be taken. However, in many cases, the cause of chronic hives is never found.

Home Remedies to Soothe Itchy Skin

If your child prefers baths to showers, a couple of tablespoons of baking soda in tepid bathwater can soothe the itch of eczema or hives. Or tie a cup of oatmeal in cheesecloth and swish it through the lukewarm bathwater until the water looks a little cloudy. You can make a traditional skin remedy by soaking ½ cup of dried camomile (or 4 camomile tea bags) in a cup of hot water for 30 minutes, straining the liquid, and adding it to a tepid bath. Cold compresses (ie, washcloths wrung out in cold water) may help to soothe an itch.

Creams and lotions made from the aloe plant are soothing to the skin. Commercial aloe products may contain only small amounts of the active extract. Instead, cut or tear the leaf of an aloe plant and rub the clear, gummy gel (not the yellow juice) on irritated skin.

Hives and angioedema can make your child extremely uncomfortable. Facial distortions caused by angioedema, in particular, can be quite visibly frightening. Although distressing, these conditions are not usually serious. Both can be triggered by any substance to which a child is allergic. Foods (eg, eggs, milk, peanuts, tree nuts) and medications, especially antibiotics, are the most frequent known and identified allergic causes. If you are certain there's a link between your child's hives or angioedema and a particular food, make every effort to keep it out of the diet. However, a definite cause or trigger for hives is often never identified. Children may suffer hives and angioedema during an otherwise mild viral infection. In rare cases, environmental or physical factors such as exposure to cold or heat may cause hives or swelling. Hives are sometimes produced or made worse by pressure, such as from tight clothes. If your child has a rash or itching along pressure lines from clothing, make sure he has comfortable, loose-fitting underwear and outerwear, including socks, belts, and shoes. Some children are vulnerable to hives and other skin troubles when they are feeling unusual emotional pressure, such as during examination time or a period of family stress.

Usually hives go away by themselves and no treatment is required. However, if symptoms persist, your pediatrician may prescribe antihistamine treatment. In most cases, treatment is required for just a short while, but sometimes antihistamines are needed daily for weeks to keep hives suppressed. Depending on your child's history and the results of allergy testing, dietary and other measures may be recommended to prevent future episodes. (For details of treatment, see Chapter 7.)

Chapter 4

Hay Fever (Allergic Rhinitis)

*T*hese are the typical symptoms and signs of allergic rhinitis, a condition commonly known as hay fever and often recognized as allergies.

- *Sneezing many times in a row*
- *Clear runny nose*
- *Blocked-up nose, mouth breathing*
- *Itching and rubbing of the nose and eyes*
- *Having to stay near the tissue box*

Mary's mom is worried about Mary starting first grade this fall. Mary's nose runs all the time with a clear, watery liquid, and she always needs to be near the tissue box. Last year in kindergarten, other children made fun of Mary because she wiped her nose so often and was constantly sniffing, making noises, and rubbing at her face and nose. Even the teacher frequently asked if Mary had a cold.

When Mary was younger, she had a constant rash that her pediatrician diagnosed as eczema. The skin condition and other symptoms, which were partly caused by an egg allergy, are much better now. However, about the time Mary's rash improved, she started having the runny, itchy nose. Mary's mother buys an over-the-counter antihistamine to give her, which helps relieve the symptoms, but it makes Mary sleepy. Sometimes she even falls asleep in class if she takes the medication before school. Mary's father understands her problems because he has hay fever, with a nose that is constantly runny and itchy during pollen season and at other times when his allergies bother him. He has also noticed that Mary wheezes when she has a cold and tends to cough whenever she runs. He knows these can be symptoms of asthma because when he was young he had asthma along with his hay fever, and he hopes that Mary doesn't develop asthma as well. Mary's parents have made an appointment with their pediatrician to evaluate all of Mary's symptoms. In particular, her father wants to talk to the pediatrician about possible treatments, as he has heard that there are now a variety of treatments for children's allergies that are a big improvement over the medications that were available when he was growing up.

. . . .

*H*ay fever (which is actually misnamed—the symptoms are not caused by hay and don't include fever) typically starts in the early school years, but it can sometimes occur as early as the second year of life. A child is more likely to develop hay fever if his parents and other family members also have allergies. The condition is more common in boys than it is in girls (almost 2:1). In children, hay fever may follow an early period in life marked by eczema and other symptoms caused by food allergy (see Chapter 3). In many cases, sneezing; nonstop runny, itchy nose; and itchy eyes set in just as eczema starts to fade.

A family history of allergies is an important factor in the development of allergic rhinitis, especially when the symptoms appear during childhood. However, the rate of hay fever, like that of asthma, appears to be increasing all over the world. The reason for this increase is not fully understood. (See "The 'Too Clean' Theory or the 'Hygiene Hypothesis'" below.)

The "Too Clean" Theory or the "Hygiene Hypothesis"

The "hygiene hypothesis," sometimes called the "too clean theory," is used to explain why there has been an increase in the number of people with allergic diseases over the last few decades in developed countries like the United States and countries of Europe, where children are growing up in a much cleaner environment than before. According to this hypothesis, 2 arms or pathways of the human immune system balance each other—one arm fights off infection, and the other arm is involved in developing allergic reactions to the environment. When the first arm is not kept busy fighting off bacteria and viruses, perhaps from an overly sanitary lifestyle, the "allergic arm" tends to becomes more active and creates allergic reactions to harmless substances like food, dust mites, mold, and pollen. Important factors likely playing a role are improved public health and hygiene, and more people receiving vaccinations to keep themselves healthy and infection-free. In this setting, the immune system has a greater tendency to go down the path of forming allergies, leading to diseases like hay fever, eczema, and asthma.

It's That Time Again

You may have come to dread a particular time of the year—usually spring or fall—because like clockwork, that's when your child's nose, eyes, mouth, and ears start to itch; he sneezes many times in a row several times a day—some doctors describe it as "machine-gun sneezing"; and his nose is stuffed up and runs with a watery discharge from morning to night. In such cases, symptoms are most often triggered by allergies to pollens and spores of seasonal plants and fungi. In most parts of the United States, trees release their pollen in the spring, grasses in the late spring and summer, and weeds—particularly ragweed, perhaps the most notorious plant allergen of all—in the early fall. Mold spores are at their highest levels and therefore are the biggest problem for people with allergies when a rainy, damp, or foggy spell is followed by a warm, dry, windy period. These conditions can occur at any time, depending on where you live. In some areas, outdoor mold levels are highest in the late summer and early fall. Fallen leaves and decaying vegetation also can lead to higher outdoor mold levels in the autumn.

The seasonal pattern of pollen release and plant growth lets you predict when symptoms are likely to appear. This helps you plan when to take whatever preventive action your pediatrician may advise to lessen the effect.

Hay Fever Symptoms Should Not Include Pain

Although at times hay fever symptoms seem to grip every part of the body in a feeling of general misery, they do not usually cause actual pain. If your child complains of pain in the face or mouth, a sensation of pressure, or headache, consult your pediatrician. The symptoms may indicate sinusitis, a dental problem, or another condition requiring treatment.

Hay Fever That Keeps Going and Going and Going

Hay fever, also known as *seasonal allergic rhinitis,* is caused by seasonal allergens (pollens). However, many people suffer from allergy symptoms all year long. This is called *perennial allergic rhinitis.* Among the typical triggers to perennial allergic rhinitis are dust mites (see Chapter 7, page 62), indoor molds, and animal dander. It's hardly surprising that allergies are so common, because all 3 are often found at high levels in many homes.

Although children with perennial allergic rhinitis may have all the usual symptoms of hay fever, for many children the most troubling symptom of year-round allergies is a constantly stuffed-up nose and difficulty breathing through the nose. Therefore, the child takes the path of least resistance, breathing with an open mouth day and night. These children may speak in an unmistakable nasal voice and often have dry, cracked lips. They tend to eat noisily. They often snore at night, have broken sleep, and wake up in the morning with a dried-out, sore throat. Postnasal drip and cough are common complaints. They frequently cough to clear their throats throughout the day. Constant mouth breathing can even end up contributing to orthodontic problems.

In the most common and uncomfortable pattern, the upper respiratory tract becomes chronically sensitized by allergens and remains so irritable that even the least irritant—perhaps a draft of cool air, air pollution, powdered ink from a photocopy, a whiff of perfume, or any strong odor—flings the child into spasms of sneezing. The nose becomes even more stuffed up and drippy. Some people have year-round allergies with seasonal worsening from pollen allergy. What's more, in many areas, the tree, grass, and weed pollen seasons last long enough to overlap, with the result that "seasonal" symptoms linger all year round.

Allergic Rhinitis and Asthma

Allergic rhinitis can stop a person from breathing through the nose, with its natural filters and air-warming system. Those with allergic rhinitis have an increased risk of asthma. One possible reason is that open-mouth breathing lets larger amounts of asthma triggers pass into the airways along with cooler, drier air, both of which can trigger asthma attacks, bringing on wheezing, coughing, and gasping for breath.

When a Cold Isn't a Cold

It's sometimes difficult to know whether the problem is hay fever or a common cold (upper respiratory infection). The diagnosis is often made when parents seek their pediatrician's advice for a lingering "cold" that their child can't shake. While symptoms of allergies and colds often overlap, there are a few telling differences. The tip-offs for hay fever are

- A clear, watery nasal discharge
- Itching of the eyes, ears, nose, or mouth
- Spasmodic sneezing

Fever is never from an allergy; it almost always suggests an infection. Antibiotics will not help allergies or a common cold from a virus. Colds or allergies can sometimes lead to ear or sinus infections; when this happens, antibiotics can be helpful. With a cold, nasal secretions are often thicker than in allergy and can be discolored (as compared with the clear, watery discharge of allergies). The child who has a cold may have a sore throat and a cough, and the child's temperature is sometimes slightly raised but not always. Itchiness is not usually a complaint with a cold, but it is the hallmark of an allergy problem. A plain old cold usually doesn't last much more than several days before it starts to get better and go away; allergy symptoms can go on for weeks to months.

Sinusitis, Ear Infections, and Allergy

As noted previously, allergic rhinitis is closely linked to sinus infections and ear infections (otitis media) in children. Several factors are involved. Respiratory allergies cause swelling and congestion in the tissues, blocking the eustachian tubes (the tiny passages that run between the ear and the back of the throat) and the openings that allow secretions to drain from the sinus cavities. Persistent blockage of the eustachian tube causes an increase in secretions from the middle ear. Germs grow in the warm, moist middle-ear environment, eventually causing an ear infection. Similarly, infections tend to develop in sinuses that are blocked and cannot drain.

Infants and young children are particularly at risk because their eustachian tubes are not as functional as those in older children and adults. Children who are exposed to secondhand cigarette smoke are also vulnerable because substances in the smoke from tobacco not only irritate the lining of the respiratory tract and stimulate it to secrete protective mucus, but also may interfere with the clearance of secretions.

Viral upper respiratory infections (in other words, colds), which are extremely common in young children, complicate allergies even more because they add further congestion and blockage. This congestion can lead to a secondary bacterial sinus infection.

Sometimes It's Fido; Sometimes Not

Furry pets are among the most common and potent causes of allergy symptoms. However, fur usually is not the only animal allergen. Even short-haired, "non-shedding" animals leave a trail of dander and saliva, as humans do. Cats are commonly more allergenic than dogs. Although certain breeds of dogs are said to be less allergenic than others, studies don't support this claim. Comparisons of dogs also show wide differences in allergenicity between individual dogs of the same breed. Reptiles, fish, and amphibians are not generally causes of allergy.

For families deeply attached to their animals, the notion of finding another home for a pet is hard to accept. Many prefer to keep the animal and battle against allergy symptoms. If you can't part with your pet, at least keep it out of your allergic child's bedroom and sweep, dust, and vacuum frequently. Another solution may be to keep your cat or dog permanently outdoors with adequate shelter. Weekly bathing in warm water has also been shown to lower the allergenic potential of pets, including animals that never venture outside. Long after an animal has left the family home, animal allergies can persist because of hair and dander left behind.

It is unwise to adopt a furry pet if you have a strong family history of allergies and, consequently, a high risk that infants and young children in your home could develop allergies. Better to wait a few years and then, if there are no signs of trouble and skin tests are clear, look into pet adoption.

A household pet may be unjustly blamed for causing allergy symptoms. Don't automatically banish Fido to the doghouse unless the results of skin testing or a specific IgE blood test (sometimes referred to as RAST; see Chapter 2, page 16) suggest that your child has an animal allergy.

Occasionally, symptoms that seem to be caused by an animal are, in fact, caused by other allergies. What happens is that pets explore outdoors, then come back into the house with a load of pollens and outdoor mold spores on their coats. Every time the hay fever sufferer pats the pets, an invisible cloud of allergens is stirred up, triggering symptoms.

With a sinus infection, nasal congestion makes it difficult for the child to breathe through the nose. The child with sinusitis often coughs at night, sleeps poorly, and consequently feels tired during the day. He may have bad breath. Sinusitis can also make asthma symptoms worse.

Quite often, chronic sinusitis—that is, a sinus infection that lasts for weeks—masquerades as year-round allergies or allergic rhinitis. Sometimes these children are thought to "always have a cold." As a result of long-standing infection, the nasal passages become persistently inflamed and irritated, with congestion similar to that seen in allergic rhinitis. There may be little or no discharge out the front of the nose if swelling has made the sinus openings too narrow to allow mucus to drain, or if the mucus runs down the back of the throat. In an older child, some pain or tenderness may be felt in the face and around the teeth, but this is not always the case. As with hay fever, symptoms such as sneezing and runny nose occur all day long, and changes or irritants in the environment can make them worse. Only when a thorough workup for allergies proves negative and the doctor finds evidence of a sinus infection does a clear picture emerge. As the infection is treated, the "allergic" or "cold" symptoms gradually resolve. In some cases, it's not only a question of allergies versus infection; both can exist at the same time. Antibiotics are prescribed to clear up bacterial ear infections and sinus infections. In some cases, your pediatrician may advise your child to be considered for ear, nose, and throat surgery, such as for removal of enlarged adenoid tissue or placement of tubes to allow ear drainage, or a procedure to drain the sinuses (also see Chapter 7, page 69). Often, when allergy-related inflammation inside the nose is properly controlled, an allergic child can avoid complications such as ear and sinus infections.

Managing Allergic Rhinitis

Pollen and Outdoor Mold
As with other types of allergies, the ideal way to manage hay fever is to find out what your child is allergic to and then avoid it. (For details about allergy testing, see Chapter 2; to read about dealing with allergies, see Chapter 7.) It sounds simple, but this is much easier said than done. To start with, many children are allergic to pollens and molds, both of which are found everywhere outdoors and cannot be completely avoided. Children need to go outside to play, so pollen exposure when outdoors is unavoidable. Exposure to outdoor pollen and mold that enters the house can be decreased by closing windows and using air conditioning, showering and changing clothes as soon as children come inside at the end of the day, and by making sure bedding is dried in a dryer, not outside on a clothes line.

Dust Mites and Molds
In addition to outdoor allergens, a child may be allergic to routinely encountered indoor substances such as dust mites or indoor molds. These everyday allergens can be kept at low levels when certain changes are made. Still, they are almost impossible to eliminate altogether, no matter how carefully you clean your home. Your child is also bound to run into indoor allergens and irritants when he ventures away from home and into other environments, such as school or friends' homes.

Dust had a reputation for causing sneezing and irritation long before allergies were called allergies. Not only does it irritate the nose, throat, and eyes, but it can also contain allergenic materials. A major cause of allergic symptoms lies beyond the dust itself. It has been traced to *dust mites*—tiny creatures that, like Dr Seuss' Whos down in Whoville, make their homes among dust specks. But whereas the Whos asked only to be left in peace, there's no getting away from dust mites. They live wherever humans live; in fact, they clean up after us. They can live on any organic debris, but their preferred diet is the half gram or so of worn-out skin cells that every human sheds daily. They also thrive on tiny fungi—like the mites, too small to be seen with the naked eye—that flourish where the relative humidity is fairly high, at 70% or more. Spores from these fungi are a major cause of allergic symptoms in humans.

Roadblock Ahead!

If your child (particularly a young child) has a runny nose with a discharge that

- Comes out of only one nostril
- Contains pus
- Smells bad
- Is tinged with blood

Don't think allergies! Instead, think that there may be an object (eg, bead, pea, pebble, part of a toy) wedged inside the nose. Call your pediatrician and don't try to remove the object yourself.

Dust mites congregate where food is plentiful. They are especially numerous in beds, pillows, upholstered furniture, and rugs. Although vacuuming and dusting can help decrease dust levels inside the home, these measures don't work very well against dust mites. As gross as it is, your child is actually allergic to a protein in dust mite feces. So steps are taken to kill dust mites and to use a containment approach to avoid mites' feces. Padded furnishings such as mattresses, box springs, pillows, and cushions should be encased in allergen-proof, zip-up covers, which are available through catalogs and specialized retailers. Covers made of non-woven synthetic fabrics are more comfortable than plastic covers and work at least as well. The microscopic dust mite fecal particles are too large to pass thorough allergy-proof covers.

Choose blankets and pillows made of synthetic materials. Because dust mites can survive in warm soapy water, wash linens weekly and other bedding, such as blankets, every 2 to 3 weeks in hot water, then put them through the hottest cycle of a clothes dryer. Pillows should be replaced every 2 or 3 years.

Allergy Shots Can Help in Hay Fever

Immunotherapy or "allergy shots"—a series of injections of allergen extracts—can bring about substantial, long-lasting relief of hay fever by desensitizing children to the effects of allergen exposure. It works by giving small but increasing doses of the substances to which a person is allergic, which gradually results in the person becoming less sensitive to the allergens (desensitization).

The procedure can be time-consuming, but when successful it can reduce symptoms and the need for medications. Immunotherapy is generally safe when carried out properly by experienced medical personnel. The most common side effects are swelling and redness at the injection site. More serious reactions, although rare, can occur, which is why allergy shots should be given in a medical office where reactions can be treated immediately. Allergy shots reduce allergen sensitivity in all parts of the body, so allergic reactions causing symptoms are suppressed in the upper and lower respiratory tract and the eyes. As a bonus, the effects of treatment can persist long after treatment has been successfully completed.

Although many effective medications are now available to treat symptoms, some people prefer to try immunotherapy. The treatment is most cost-effective in those who are sensitive to airborne allergens such as pollens. It is also more effective if steps are first taken to reduce exposure to environmental allergens such as dust mites and animal dander, especially in the home.

Dust mites also abound in cuddly stuffed toys. When possible, replace soft, plush-covered toys with others that have smooth plastic bodies and washable clothes. If your child has a favorite soft toy from which she can't be parted, wash it every other day or so in hot water and dry it at the highest setting. Or seal soft toys in plastic bags and put them in the freezer for at least 5 hours or overnight once a week. Dust mites cannot survive longer than 5 hours at freezing temperature; you can then rinse the toys in warm water and put them in the dryer to get rid of the dead mites. These steps will not necessarily remove all of the allergenic dust mite feces, but they help!

Keep bulky fabrics and dust-catching clutter out of your child's room. Remove wall-to-wall carpeting, if possible. Floors should be wooden, tile, or vinyl—anything but carpet. Damp mopping and electrostatic floor mops are helpful for clean up. If you prefer rugs for comfort, use small cotton or synthetic throw rugs that can be washed weekly in hot water. Curtains should be easily washable.

When it comes to the walls, the aim is to eliminate horizontal surfaces that trap dust. There should be no picture frames or shelves displaying books or ornaments, and all surfaces—on dressers, bedside tables, and other furniture—should be easy to wipe clean.

Avoid humidifiers and vaporizers. Dust mites need humidity to live, and humidification will only further help the mite population grow. For the same reason, using a dehumidifier in certain moist geographical locations can be beneficial by helping to keep the humidity below the range that suits mites and molds. However, if you use a dehumidifier, it's essential not only to empty the water pan but also to scour it daily to prevent the growth of invisible molds. High-efficiency particulate air (HEPA) cleaning devices are useful for getting rid of some airborne allergens but are not generally useful for dust mites. (For a more detailed discussion, see Chapter 12.)

No matter how careful you may be, you can't protect a child as if she were a hothouse plant. And even if you were to succeed in eliminating most environmental allergens in your home, children still get exposed at school and at playmates' homes. Furthermore, it's hard to avoid the normally harmless kinds of nonallergenic irritants that can set off symptoms in a nose already primed and twitchy from allergen exposure.

Medications

Long experience has shown that antihistamines are effective medications for relieving sneezing, itching, and runny nose caused by seasonal hay fever and perennial allergic rhinitis. (For details about allergy medications, see Chapter 7). Many older-type antihistamines available without prescription may cause drowsiness; your pediatrician may want to avoid recommending them or advise they only be used at night. Newer antihistamines (eg, loratadine, cetirizine, levocetirizine, fexofenadine) are much less likely to cause sleepiness. Some are available without a prescription. These are more often recommended because of their better safety profile. There are antihistamines also now available that are sprayed directly into the nose and have similar or sometimes better results than when given by mouth. Antihistamine therapy, whether by mouth or by spray, is most helpful for the runny nose, itching, and sneezing symptoms of allergic rhinitis and less helpful for nasal congestion.

Decongestants are often prescribed together with antihistamines to unblock the nose in children with allergic rhinitis. However, oral decongestants can have a number of side effects, making children feel overexcited and shaky or jittery. These medications should be used very sparingly and only as recommended by your pediatrician. Decongestants can be given as a nasal spray or nose drops, but if they are used too long in this form, they can have a rebound effect, making the nose even more congested and irritated. This condition, called *rhinitis medicamentosa,* is harder to treat than the original stuffy nose.

Corticosteroids given as a nasal spray are currently the most effective medications available for reducing nasal inflammation and congestion. They act by relieving and preventing the symptoms of year-round or seasonal allergies. When used carefully, these medications often give better results than all other forms of medication treatment for allergic disease. Your pediatrician will prescribe the lowest-possible dose to control the symptoms. Your pediatrician will closely monitor your child's progress to avoid side effects and may recommend, at some point, a decrease in your child's dose or even a complete break in the treatment. (See Chapter 7 for details about treatments for allergy-related problems).

Chapter 5

Food Allergies

An estimated 1 in 20 children has a food allergy. Food allergies can be severe, requiring strict avoidance of the triggering food(s) and prompt treatment of any allergic reaction. Foods can also trigger a variety of symptoms that are not classic allergies. It is important to seek a diagnosis so your child can safely enjoy nutritious foods that are not a problem and avoid foods that cause symptoms.

At child care, 2-year-old Justin is given a cracker with peanut butter by a fellow preschooler who wants to share. It is the first time Justin has ever eaten peanuts or peanut butter. Within 5 minutes of eating just a small amount, Justin develops swelling around his mouth and hives all over his body. The school administrator calls Justin's mother, who arrives at school, gives him an antihistamine, and takes him to an urgent care center where he is checked and said to be wheezing. The doctors give him an epinephrine (adrenaline) injection and Justin feels better quickly. Later that day, Justin's pediatrician examines him and orders a blood test to check for peanut allergy. The test comes back strongly positive, meaning that Justin is allergic to peanuts. The pediatrician advises that Justin must strictly avoid peanuts and prescribes an epinephrine (adrenaline) auto-injection device for Justin's mother to keep with her at all times in case Justin ever accidentally eats peanut products. Justin's mother also orders a medical identification bracelet for him to wear at all times that identifies him as having severe peanut allergy. Everyone at the child care center is alerted to make sure that Justin is never given peanut products. His mother decides to eliminate peanut butter from their home when she learns that even a small amount left on a knife could end up contaminating Justin's food and cause a serious reaction. With some education and preparation, Justin's family learns that they can keep him safe and healthy, allowing him to do everything the other children do except for eating peanut products.

....

*A*lthough many people use "food allergy" and "food intolerance" interchangeably, the terms describe 2 different conditions. *Food allergy* occurs when the immune system, designed to fight infection, mistakenly attacks food proteins. The most common type of immune reaction leading to food allergy is when the individual's immune system forms specific IgE antibodies against the food protein. Each time the allergic person eats the problem food and the food protein comes in contact with the IgE made against it, certain chemicals such as histamine are released that cause hives, itching, swelling, wheezing, and other allergy symptoms.

Food intolerance is a general term usually used to refer to a food-induced reaction that does not involve the immune system. Lactose-intolerance is a well-known example. People with lactose intolerance don't make enough lactase, an enzyme that is needed to digest lactose, the sugar in milk. When lactose-intolerant people drink milk or eat milk-based foods, they have symptoms affecting the digestive tract, such as gas, bloating, stomachache, and diarrhea. This is not the same as a food allergy.

Food Allergy Symptoms

Symptoms of a food allergy reaction can include vomiting, diarrhea, an itchy rash (ranging from just around the mouth and face to total-body hives), mouth and throat itchiness and swelling, difficulty breathing, and wheezing. Most true food allergy reactions occur within minutes after ingesting the food. In some cases, chronic symptoms such as persistent itchy skin rashes, eczema, or chronic gut symptoms (eg, vomiting, pain, poor growth) are the result of food allergy.

The intensity of an allergic reaction may range from mild to severe at different times, partly depending on how much of an allergenic food your child eats. However, certain highly allergic children need to swallow only a very small amount of an offending food to have a serious allergic reaction. Some foods are more likely than others to cause severe reactions, such as peanut, tree nuts, and seafood. Your child's general health may influence the severity of the allergy. Children with asthma are at higher risk for severe reactions. Although food allergy can cause severe reactions, fatalities are rare and often attributed to delay in appropriate treatment. For those with potentially severe food allergy (anaphylaxis) it is important to learn how to strictly avoid the trigger food, and understand how to recognize and promptly treat a severe allergic reaction.

Diagnosing Food Allergies

As with all forms of allergy, your pediatrician will review your child's medical history, question you closely about the foods she eats, and review your family's medical history for allergy-related conditions. Your pediatrician may also order a blood test to detect allergic antibodies to specific suspected foods (see Chapter 2), or send your child to an allergist for allergy skin testing or additional tests. The specific allergy IgE blood tests and skin tests provide valuable information; however, one may be preferable in some circumstances. For example, your physician may order a blood test rather than skin testing if there is a skin disease or a rash that makes skin testing difficult. Your pediatrician also may order a blood test if antihistamine drugs (a class of medications that blunt allergy skin test reactions, making testing not possible) cannot be stopped before skin testing.

If your child has frequent symptoms that may or may not be food related, your pediatrician may also ask you to keep a food diary (see Chapter 2, page 17), noting every food your child eats, together with any symptoms that occur. If symptoms seem to be linked to a particular food, you may be advised to keep it out of your child's diet to see if symptoms improve, or additional allergy tests might be ordered to evaluate the suspected food. Even though the results of skin tests or specific IgE blood tests may help indicate a potential allergy, positive results do not always mean that your child is definitely allergic to the food. Positive results must be interpreted by a professional experienced in diagnosing allergy using all available clinical information. The pediatrician or allergist will consider the test result (including the degree of the positive result) along with clues from your child's history to determine if there is an allergy. In fact, a skin test or blood test may continue to give a positive result for a time after the child has outgrown that allergy. In some cases, especially with allergies that primarily affect the gut, tests can be negative even though there is an allergy. Sometimes a physician, usually an allergist, has to watch your child eat the food gradually and monitor whether there are symptoms; this test is called a *food challenge* or medically supervised feeding test. This is sometimes the only way to confirm an allergy or to know whether the allergy has resolved for follow-up.

Managing Food Allergies

There are currently no cures for a food allergy. Management is based on avoiding the food and being prepared to treat an allergic reaction should the food be eaten accidentally. Antihistamines can help mild symptoms such as itching and hives, but an epinephrine injection is necessary for severe symptoms or breathing difficulties (eg, throat swelling, wheezing). If epinephrine needs to be given, the child should be immediately taken for emergency medical care, or if necessary, 911 called. (See Chapter 7.)

If your pediatrician believes there is any risk that your child could have a severe allergic reaction (an anaphylactic reaction) to food (see chapters 1 and 6), your pediatrician will recommend that you—and your child, when old enough to use it by himself—always carry an epinephrine autoinjector device in case of an accidental ingestion of the food. It is essential that you review with your doctor how and when to use this medication. The devices are easy to use and the medication is safe, but it is important to be familiar with the device being prescribed so that there are no delays in providing emergency treatment. A child at risk for anaphylaxis should also wear medical identification. For details about allergy treatments and prevention, see Chapter 7.

Food Allergy Myths and Misconceptions

1. *Food allergy affects behavior.* There is no convincing research results showing that a true food allergy causes problems such as attention-deficit/hyperactivity disorder or autism. Some studies show that chemical preservatives or dyes, presumably through a pharmacologic rather than allergic mechanism, might contribute to these problems, but the evidence is weak and not widely accepted by experts.

2. *Sugar allergy causes behavioral problems.* Parents may blame high-sugar foods for unusual behavior. However, the results of several carefully controlled studies of preschool and school-aged children showed sugar or artificial sweeteners had no effect on behavior.

3. *Each allergic reaction gets worse.* It is not automatically the case that each subsequent exposure to the food will result in a worse allergic reaction. The severity of a subsequent reaction is not easily predicted and can be worse, the same, or milder than previous reactions.

4. *Peanut-allergic children should avoid all kinds of nuts.* Peanut is a legume and *not* of the tree nuts family. Many children with peanut allergy can tolerate tree nuts, and vice versa. However, some children can be allergic to multiple different foods, including peanut and certain tree nuts. Make sure you are clear what the situation is with your child.

There's only one sure way to prevent food allergy symptoms, and that's to avoid the problem food altogether, in all forms, at all times. Sometimes this is easier said than done. Product labels must be read carefully each time to ensure the allergic food is not an ingredient. Read the label each time because ingredients may change. This is extremely important for patients with severe food allergy. At home, avoid cross-contact of safe foods with an allergen. For example, a knife used in peanut butter and then in jelly may leave peanut residue in the jelly jar that could cause a reaction when the jelly is used another day. Similarly, be careful when preparing foods and using cutting boards, mixing spoons, and heating surfaces. In restaurants, have a careful conversation with the waiter to be sure that the allergen is not an ingredient or contaminant of your child's meal, although this may not be guaranteed. For school, bringing safe foods from home may avoid problems with cafeteria meals, although many schools can provide safe foods with proper preparation. Strict no-sharing policies must be followed to prevent accidental ingestions. Also avoid using food products in craft and science projects to steer clear of accidental exposures.

Read Labels!

US labeling laws require disclosure of peanut, tree nuts (eg, almond, hazelnut, walnut), milk, egg, wheat, soy, fish, and crustacean shellfish ingredients in packaged manufactured foods. When a tree nut, fish, or crustacean shellfish is an ingredient, the type must be disclosed (eg, walnut, cod, shrimp).

Additional foods (eg, sesame) are being considered for inclusion in labeling laws.

Manufacturers may voluntarily indicate if an allergen is a potential unintended contaminant of a food by using advisory label terms such as "may contain" or "prepared in a facility that processes." These voluntary statements cannot be used to know how much of an allergen is in a food or how often a food may contain the unintended allergen. Therefore, to play it safe, these foods are best avoided.

If your child is allergic to a food not covered by the law, you have to be extra careful. For example, there is a chance it is an ingredient in descriptive terms such as "spices."

In some cases, you may need to contact a manufacturer to get additional information about ingredients. Whenever in doubt, just avoid that food.

It's a fairly simple matter to keep a problem food away from a very young child who eats meals and snacks under the watchful eye of parents or caregivers. However, it is more difficult with an older child who has less supervision while eating. Not only your child but also his friends and their parents should understand how serious the condition is and how important it is to avoid the allergen in any form. Above all, children should be warned never to share or taste another child's food.

Be sure to provide full information about your child's food allergy to school and camp personnel and child care providers. Update information regularly at the start of each school year and as new facts become available. In this regard, it is important to report accurate information, ie, definite food allergies, not minor food sensitivities.

The Food Allergy & Anaphylaxis Network for Up-to-date Information

The Food Allergy & Anaphylaxis Network (FAAN), a nonprofit organization, was established to increase awareness about food allergies and provide unbiased information and support for people with food allergies. The organization's main focus is on children because food allergies are much more common in children than in adults. The FAAN provides a variety of educational materials that may make it easier to approach your child's school.

Contact the FAAN at www.foodallergy.org or 800/929-4040.

Food Allergies May Go Away With Time

Many children outgrow food allergies after a period of strict avoidance varying from months to years. More than 85% of allergies to milk, egg, wheat, and soy resolve during childhood, often before school age. Only about 1 in 5 children, on the other hand, ever outgrow a peanut allergy. Allergies to fish, shellfish, and tree nuts also tend to be more persistent, but some children outgrow these as well. Repeat allergy testing may be done at some point on your child for the food that formerly caused problems to see if the food allergy has resolved. It is important to regularly follow up with your pediatrician or allergist to discuss management and the possibility that the food allergy has resolved. Never try to intentionally test your child by feeding an allergen at home! If follow-up skin or blood test results are favorable, your doctor may suggest a medically supervised cautious feeding (also known as a food challenge) to see if the allergy has disappeared.

Preventing Allergies Through Diet

For infants at risk for allergy (eg, newborn with parent or sibling with a documented allergy), there are a couple of things that reduce the risk of or delay allergic problems such as eczema.

1. Breastfeed exclusively for at least 4 to 6 months.

2. If unable to breastfeed or if supplementing in the first months, use a low-allergen formula such as an extensively hydrolyzed or partially hydrolyzed formula rather than a regular cow's-milk formula or soy-based formula.

Studies have not been conclusive about the effectiveness of refraining from eating specific foods during pregnancy or lactation, or waiting extensive periods before introducing potentially allergenic foods to an otherwise healthy infant. Further research is underway to clarify this important issue.

Common Food Allergens

Any food may cause an allergic reaction, but 90% of food allergies in children are caused by just 6 common foods or food groups—milk, eggs, peanuts, tree nuts, soy, and wheat. In adults, a similar percentage of serious allergies are caused by just 4 foods—peanuts, tree nuts, fish, and shellfish. Allergies to fruits and vegetables are much less common and usually less severe.

Cow's Milk

Allergy to cow's milk is among the most common hypersensitivity in young children, probably because it is the first foreign protein that many infants ingest in such a large quantity, especially if they are bottle-fed. If there is a cow's-milk allergy, occasionally even a breastfed infant may have colic or eczema until milk and dairy foods are eliminated from the mother's diet. Between 2 and 3 out of every 100 children younger than 3 years have allergy symptoms linked to cow's milk.

Vomiting after feeding is the most common way a child shows a milk allergy, but more severe reactions can occur. Colic, crying, and gassiness can sometimes be the only manifestation of cow's-milk allergy in very young infants. (It must be said, though, that in the great majority of infants, no cause for colic is ever found, and the inconsolable crying eventually stops without treatment, never to return, before the baby is 6 months old). Other early and more subtle symptoms of milk allergy often involve the itchy, dry rash of eczema (atopic dermatitis; see Chapter 3). Of course the most obvious kind of reaction to milk is when the child drinks milk or eats a milk product and immediately develops breathing problems or hives. Most children with cow's-milk allergy are also allergic to milk from goats or sheep, so these are not good substitutes.

Soy-based formula may or may not be suitable for milk-allergic infants because some who are sensitive to cow's milk are also unable to tolerate soy protein. If your cow's-milk–allergic baby does not tolerate soy formula, your pediatrician may recommend a special formula made of extensively hydrolyzed protein or an amino acid elemental formula.

Many children outgrow milk allergy as their immune systems mature. However, your pediatrician will probably suggest that allergy tests be performed before your child tries milk again. If testing shows the allergy has gone away, milk can be cautiously given to your child in gradually increasing amounts in the doctor's office, where any reaction can be monitored and if necessary, treated. If your child simply has lactose intolerance (see page 49), allergy testing is usually unnecessary, and milk and milk products can be gradually reintroduced at home while you watch for symptoms. In supermarkets, there are products with varying reduced content of the sugar lactose that help children with lactose intolerance to be able to have milk in their diet.

Milk and foods derived from milk are important sources of *calcium,* a mineral essential for strong bones and teeth, muscle and nerve function, and the health of every system in the body. Dark-green leafy vegetables, canned fish eaten with the bones (eg, sardines, salmon), calcium-fortified orange juice, dried figs and prunes, tofu, and dried beans are among the many rich nondairy sources of calcium for older children who cannot tolerate milk, cheese, and yogurt.

Eggs
Children who are allergic to eggs are reacting primarily to the protein in the egg white. However, because egg yolk can often be contaminated with egg white, it's safer for egg-allergic children to avoid egg altogether. Luckily, while eggs are nutritionally valuable and an excellent source of protein, they are not essential for good nutrition. Meat, fish, dairy products, grains, and legumes are excellent alternative sources of similar protein, minerals, and vitamins. If your child is allergic to eggs, watch out for hidden egg ingredients such as an egg-based glaze on top of certain breads or egg used to hold breading on fried food.

Egg substitutes developed for low-cholesterol diets cannot be used. They are cholesterol-free (because they do not contain yolk, the part of the egg where the cholesterol is found) but still contain egg protein because they are made with egg white, the part responsible for causing allergies. Some vaccines may contain egg proteins and should be avoided or taken with caution by those with severe egg allergy. The measles-mumps-rubella vaccine is considered safe for those with egg allergy, but talk to your doctor about seasonal influenza vaccines and others that may have egg proteins.

Peanuts and Tree Nuts

When is a nut not a nut? When it's a legume—like peanuts, which are cousins to peas and beans. Because peanuts and tree nuts come from different plant families, a child who is sensitive to peanuts can often eat walnuts, pecans, and other tree nuts without a problem. However, caution is needed because peanut-allergic children, for unknown reasons, are more likely also to have a separate tree-nut allergy.

Like eggs, peanuts are delicious and nutritious but not essential for a healthy diet. No nutritional substitutes are needed. Most people with a peanut allergy tolerate other legumes such as soy and beans, even when sometimes skin or blood tests will come up positive for these other legumes.

Peanuts, although generally pretty easy to avoid, can sometimes show up in foods when least expected. Peanuts are often ground up and used as bulking agents in food products such as candies. Peanut butter is sometimes used by restaurants and caterers as a "glue" in food preparation to hold the food item together. Therefore, it is imperative that you not only read labels carefully to make sure peanuts are not unsuspected ingredients in commercial foods, but that you also question and clarify the content of food being bought and eaten at restaurants, or prepared and consumed at locations other than your own house.

Allergy to tree nuts—walnuts, pecans, cashews, Brazil nuts, almonds, hazel nuts; all the nuts in hard shells—can be as severe as peanut allergy, and the same warnings apply. One child may have an allergy to only one tree nut, while another may have an allergy to a number of tree nuts. Confusion can sometimes occur about the different types of tree nuts, so tree-nut–allergic individuals often just stay away from all of them, to play it safe. Make caregivers, teachers, friends, and family members aware that your child must strictly avoid all products with even a trace of nuts and peanuts because nut allergy, in general, is the most severe of all the food allergies.

Soy

Babies fed soy formula, like that of cow's milk, can develop a rash, runny nose, wheezing, diarrhea, or vomiting from allergy to the soy protein. When changing to a soy formula, some infants who are allergic to cow's milk are found to also be allergic to soy. If this is the case, your pediatrician may recommend a low-allergenic formula made with extensively hydrolyzed protein or amino acid elemental formula. Children with soy allergy generally tolerate soy oil because it contains minimal protein. Soy lecithin is a fatty derivative of soy that is extremely low in soy protein and usually tolerated by those with a soy allergy.

> **Food Allergy Notes**
>
> - If your child has symptoms indicating allergy after being given a particular food, keep it out of the diet and discuss the symptoms with your pediatrician.
>
> - Some children with milk or egg allergy may tolerate a small amount of milk or egg if it is cooked into a baked good such as bread or a muffin. However, other children react to even this small, extensively heated amount.
>
> - A child avoiding multiple foods because of food allergy could be at risk of malnutrition. Discuss seeing a registered dietitian with your doctor, to be able to get some expert help about how to wisely feed your child who has significant dietary restrictions.
>
> - Your child with a food allergy should be able to do every activity another child can do except eat the food to which she is allergic. Talk with your pediatrician or allergist about allergen avoidance, as well as dietary and treatment strategies to maintain a safe and healthy lifestyle.

Wheat and Gluten

Rice and oats are usually the first cereals introduced into the diet because they are less likely than other grains to cause allergy problems. If there are no problems with oats, wheat is given next. Wheat is the grain most often associated with allergies, but even so, it is still an uncommon food allergy. This is fortunate because wheat is found in so many prepared foods.

There are 2 types of negative immune reactions to wheat. The first is classic food allergy, with symptoms such as hives or wheezing that occur immediately after the child eats a food made with wheat. The second is called *celiac disease.* Gluten is a protein found in grains such as wheat, rye, and barley. In a sensitive child, gluten damages the lining of the small intestine and interferes with nutrient absorption. This damage can go undetected for some time. Typical symptoms of celiac disease are abdominal pain, diarrhea, irritability, poor weight gain, and slow growth. Celiac disease may reveal itself shortly after the infant has his first bowl of cereal, but in some cases, symptoms are so minor that the condition can smolder at a low level for years and a diagnosis may not be made until adolescence or even adulthood.

Lactose Intolerance

Lactose intolerance is not an allergy; it's a digestive problem—an inability to digest *lactose,* the sugar in milk. People with lactose intolerance have low levels of an enzyme, lactase, which is normally produced in the lining of the small intestine. When there is not enough lactase enzyme to break down lactose into forms that can be easily absorbed, the milk sugar ferments in the intestine, causing cramps, bloating, gas (flatulence), diarrhea, and nausea anywhere from about 30 minutes to 2 hours after a meal. The symptoms of lactose intolerance are never serious or life-threatening, but they can be uncomfortable.

If lactose intolerance is suspected as the cause of your child's symptoms, your pediatrician will likely suggest that your child try a lactose-free milk and avoid all foods that contain cow's milk (eg, cheeses). Tests to prove this condition are rarely needed. Improvement on a lactose-free diet, in itself, helps prove the diagnosis. Lactose intolerance is common in older children and adults, particularly in certain ethnic populations (eg, Eskimos, Asians, American Indians, African Americans). Symptoms of lactose intolerance are fairly easy to manage with dietary measures. Most supermarkets sell lactose-reduced milk and foods that can substitute for cow's milk and cow's-milk products. Lactase enzyme tablets or liquid are available that can be added to milk at home to reduce the lactose content by about 70%. Chewable tablets taken before a meal are available to help digest solid foods that contain lactose.

A young child with lactose intolerance should avoid not only milk but also foods containing milk, including yogurt, ice cream, and cheese. If milk is ruled out altogether for the child, your pediatrician will suggest alternative sources for calcium, like for children with cow's-milk allergy. Certain less-sensitive children can usually eat small amounts of lactose-containing foods. Many children can enjoy limited quantities of chocolate milk or aged cheeses and fresh frozen yogurts, where lactose is naturally broken down in the manufacturing process. As time goes on, you and your child will be able to gauge by trial and error the amount of milk or milk-based foods he can handle.

Chapter 6

Killer Allergies: Anaphylaxis

*A*naphylaxis *is the most intense form of allergic reaction but luckily, also the rarest. It comes on without warning, causes severe symptoms, and may lead to death unless treated. Anaphylaxis is always an emergency and requires immediate medical attention.*

Twelve-year-old Bryan likes to play around the ice plant in his backyard, a spot that also attracts many bees. One day, when running barefoot, Bryan is stung on his foot by a bee. Soon afterward he develops mild hives over most of his body and has some swelling in the area of the sting. His mother calls their pediatrician, who tells her to give the youngster an antihistamine and come to the office. Bryan responds so well—the hives quickly go away—that she decides not to bother to go in.

A few days later, Bryan is stung on the hand. Right away he goes into the house to find his mother. His chest feels tight, he is wheezing, and his throat feels swollen and itchy. His mother immediately takes him to the nearest hospital emergency department, where he is treated with epinephrine (adrenaline) and given antihistamine intravenously so the medication can be quickly absorbed.

When Bryan's symptoms are under control, the emergency medicine physician explains that the attack was a severe form of allergy known as *anaphylaxis* and prescribes preloaded epinephrine autoinjectors—a couple for Bryan's mother to keep in the house and the car, and another for Bryan to carry with him at all times in case he is stung again.

At a follow-up appointment, the pediatrician refers Bryan for evaluation by an allergy specialist. The results of allergy skin testing show that Bryan is highly allergic to honeybee venom. The allergy specialist makes sure that Bryan and his parents all know exactly how and when to use the epinephrine autoinjector. The doctor also recommends that Bryan start allergy shots (immunotherapy) to desensitize him to bee venom.

*A*naphylaxis, like less-severe forms of allergy, is a rare overreaction by the immune system to invasion by a foreign allergen. But while less-severe allergies may affect one or more body systems and occur more or less gradually, such as when a child has eczema on the skin or wheezing in the airways, anaphylaxis can take over every system at once with sudden, full-force symptoms.

Within minutes of being exposed to an allergen, a youngster in the throes of anaphylaxis may turn bright red, break out in hives, and have marked swelling (angioedema; see Chapter 3, page 28) of the face, especially the lips and eyes, and inside the mouth, throat, and voice box. The reaction causes the smooth muscles of the airways of the lungs—these are involuntary muscles—to go into spasm, closing down the airways. The child wheezes as she gasps for breath. Her pulse races and her skin turns clammy. She may be overcome by nausea, vomiting, and diarrhea. In severe anaphylaxis, her blood vessels relax, preventing the heart from maintaining normal blood pressure, and the child goes into shock.

Emergency Help for Anaphylaxis

If you suspect your child is having anaphylaxis (he's suddenly weak, pale, and short of breath and has a rash or widespread swelling), call Emergency Medical Services (911 in most areas) immediately. If your child stops breathing or you can't feel a pulse, start cardiopulmonary resuscitation (CPR) as soon as you have called for help.

An identical type of sudden, rare reaction can occur that does not involve the IgE allergy antibodies (see Chapter 1, page 5). This is called an *anaphylactoid reaction,* which means that it is like anaphylaxis, though caused by a different mechanism. It may come on during exercise, or when a susceptible youngster takes certain medications, such as aspirin or another nonsteroidal anti-inflammatory drug (NSAID). The symptoms are the same as those of anaphylaxis and an attack requires the same prompt emergency measures.

Researchers believe that, in general, the sooner symptoms appear, the more severe an attack of anaphylaxis is likely to be. In some cases, an attack occurs in 2 phases. Treatment is given and the symptoms clear up, only to have symptoms reappear with the same intensity after a lapse of several hours. The physician treating a child for anaphylaxis will keep her under observation or warn caregivers to watch her carefully until the danger period has passed.

Few Children Are at Risk

Many substances have the potential to cause anaphylaxis, but the chances of your child having an anaphylactic reaction are quite remote. However, this severe type of allergic reaction is something everyone should be able to recognize, so as to know when to get emergency help, whether for your own child or somebody else's.

Risk Factors for Anaphylaxis

Unless a youngster has previously had a warning episode with severe allergic symptoms, it's impossible to foresee when anaphylaxis may strike. However, there are certain conditions or risk factors—even if they don't actually cause anaphylaxis—that tend to be found more often in those who experience attacks. They are warning signals to watch for.

Allergies

Although anaphylaxis or an anaphylactoid reaction can occur in a person with no previously identified allergies (such as to penicillin or bee stings), generally, people who experience anaphylaxis are more likely to have a history of allergies than the general population.

Type of Allergen

For undetermined reasons, certain allergens are more often involved in anaphylaxis. Food (eg, peanuts, milk, eggs, tree nuts) and insect venom (especially bee) are the leading causes of anaphylactic reactions among children. Much less common causes are antibiotics (eg, penicillin) and latex. These same allergens plus shellfish are frequent causes in adults; shellfish causes fewer problems in children, possibly because children eat shellfish less often. When a youngster is allergic to medication—commonly, an antibiotic in the penicillin family—the risk of anaphylaxis is higher if the dose is given by injection, rather than by mouth.

Frequency of Contact

The risk of anaphylaxis seems to be higher when a youngster has had several brief exposures to an allergenic substance, followed by a long contact-free lull. The next contact after this interval is the one that may trip the wire for an anaphylactic episode. The more often a person comes in contact with a potentially allergenic substance, the higher the statistical chances that an anaphylactic reaction could occur. But as noted previously, anaphylaxis is highly unpredictable and an attack may occur in the rare child who has no previous known contact with the allergen.

Previous Severity of Attack

Children who had a severe reaction in the past are at higher risk for another severe attack than children who had a milder reaction. However, even children who have had only minor problems in the past can still go on to have a life-threatening episode given the right circumstances; one always has to be on guard.

Causes of Anaphylaxis

Although almost any substance could cause anaphylaxis, the leading anaphylaxis triggers in children have been narrowed down to the following 3 categories:

- Foods
- Insect stings and bites
- Medications (least common)

> ### Keep Your Child's School Informed About Anaphylaxis
>
> Let teachers and school personnel know if your child is severely allergic and is at risk for anaphylaxis. Make sure teachers know what symptoms to look for and what measures to take. An epinephrine autoinjector should be kept in the school office or, if the child is old enough, with the student. Talk to the school nurse to make sure he or she is familiar with emergency measures for anaphylaxis.

Foods

Peanuts, milk, eggs, and tree nuts are the most common food triggers for childhood allergy (see Chapter 5) and anaphylaxis. Peanuts are a leading cause of anaphylaxis in all age groups in the United States, and peanut allergy, unlike egg and milk allergies, is rarely outgrown. Because peanuts are legumes, related to peas and beans but not to tree nuts, a child who is allergic to peanuts is not necessarily allergic to tree nuts and may be able to eat them. However, there is a danger that peanuts may sometimes be snuck in with tree nuts. Parents and children who are allergic to peanuts or tree nuts need to read food labels carefully and be aware that nuts are hidden ingredients in many foods (see Chapter 5, page 48, and Appendix A).

Milk and foods containing milk protein are often the cause of anaphylaxis among babies and toddlers because milk is such an important part of their diet. Egg can initiate anaphylaxis but is less likely to be the cause compared with peanuts, tree nuts, and milk. Although egg white is the main allergy and anaphylaxis trigger in egg-allergic children, a youngster who is highly allergic should avoid yolks as well because they may be contaminated by traces of protein from the white.

Sometimes it's difficult to know which food set off a severe reaction. Your pediatrician may use a specific IgE blood test (ie, RAST) or refer your child for skin tests (see Chapter 2) to identify your child's food allergies.

Insect Stings and Bites

The risk of an allergic reaction to an insect sting has been known, if not understood, for a very long time. Almost 5,000 years ago, scribes recorded the death of an Egyptian king who collapsed after a wasp or hornet sting. Insect stings commonly cause local pain and swelling whether your child is allergic or not. A child with venom allergy has more than just local discomfort and skin changes to the sting; that child can break out in hives, wheeze, and develop anaphylaxis.

Honeybees are the main offenders; hornets, yellow jackets, and wasps can also deliver a potentially lethal sting resulting in a severe allergic reaction (anaphylaxis). Fire ants are a growing problem, especially in the South and Southwest. Deerflies and some other biting insects have rarely been linked to anaphylaxis. However, although bites from houseflies, mosquitoes, fleas, and ticks can cause symptoms ranging from a mild, itchy nuisance to Lyme disease (a potentially serious disorder caused by germs carried by deer ticks), they almost never lead to life-threatening allergic reactions.

When to Get Help

Your child may have pain and swelling after an insect sting, but there is no cause for alarm as long as the reaction stays localized to the site of the sting. Hives that occur immediately after an insect sting may warrant seeking medical help, but as long as there are no other serious symptoms such as breathing difficulties, the child usually does just fine. However, if your child has skin symptoms plus problems in another part of the body (eg, wheezing, hoarseness, a swelling sensation inside the mouth or throat), call Emergency Medical Services (911 in most areas) at once. The results of anaphylaxis are so serious that when in doubt, doctors always treat rather than wait and see.

Even if anaphylaxis does not develop, report severe or unusual symptoms to your pediatrician, who may refer your child to a pediatric allergy specialist to perform allergy tests to identify or confirm your child's sensitivity.

If your doctor believes there is a risk of anaphylaxis, your doctor will prescribe an epinephrine (adrenaline) autoinjector for you (and your child when she is old enough to use it) to carry at all times and will tell you how to use it in emergencies. Your child should wear a medical identification tag specifying what she is allergic to.

Allergy Shots for Insect Stings

If the results of tests show that your child has an insect sting allergy, your pediatrician may recommend allergy shots (venom immunotherapy), which give good protection against future reactions.

Venom immunotherapy enables the insect-allergic child to develop immunity to the insect venom, preventing the venom from setting off the child's allergic mechanisms. This reduces the risk that the child will have a serious allergic reaction after future insect stings.

The treatment is given by injecting gradually stronger doses of insect venom into the child's arm over an extended period. Injections are given once or twice a week at first, then at longer intervals. When the venom strength has reached a predetermined goal, the child gets a maintenance injection once a month to keep up a good level of protection (see also Chapter 7).

Protect Your Child From Insect Stings

- For outside play, dress your insect-allergic child in a long-sleeved shirt, long pants, and shoes and socks when you can. A broad-brimmed hat can help to keep insects away from the face.

- Make sure your child wears shoes; kids are often stung on the bottom of a bare foot.

- Avoid bright-colored clothes, perfume, or aftershave lotion, which can attract insects.

- Apply insect repellent to your child's clothing, not the skin. Read the label to check that repellent contains no more than 10% DEET. DEET is effective but can be harmful when absorbed through the skin.

- Oils of citronella and peppermint are natural insect repellents that can be mixed with vegetable oil and applied to clothing.

- Keep door and window screens in good repair.

- When outside, warn your child to avoid areas that attract flying insects, such as beds of flowers and succulents such as ice plant, flowering shrubs, fruit trees and bushes, and garbage containers.

- When eating outside, such as at picnics, check fruits and sweet foods for insects. Look inside cans and bottles before drinking.

Medications

Many different medications have been linked to anaphylaxis attacks. It's not surprising that penicillin and some related antibiotics are often implicated because bacterial infections requiring antibiotic treatment are among the most frequent childhood illnesses. Some children who are allergic to penicillin may also have an allergic cross-reaction when given one of a related group of antibiotics, the cephalosporins, although such cross-reactions are rare. Anaphylaxis can occur no matter how a medication is given but happens more often after injections.

Bee Sting and Penicillin Allergies Don't Seem to Run in Families

Although a tendency toward developing allergies, in general, runs in many families, family history and genetics do not seem to be important in developing a specific allergy to penicillin or bee stings. In other words, although either parent may have had a severe allergic reaction to a bee sting or to treatment with amoxicillin (an antibiotic related to penicillin), the child does not have an increased risk of having a bad reaction to that specific agent. The tendency toward developing a specific allergy, unlike allergies in general, does not appear to run in families.

Unless your child has a proven sensitivity to penicillin or another medication, there is little need to worry about the possibility of a reaction. Most medications are safe, and a serious reaction is unlikely to happen more than once in several million doses.

> **Many Side Effects of Medications Are Not Symptoms of an Allergy**
> Stomach upset or loose stools are sometimes a side effect of antibiotic treatment but usually not an allergic reaction by themselves. If you have difficulty telling normal side effects from allergy symptoms, ask your pediatrician to explain the difference. If your child has any unusual reaction after taking medication, call your pediatrician at once.

Your pediatrician keeps a record of your child's allergies on file but will always ask about medication allergies before writing a prescription. There are usually several effective alternatives for any medication that your child cannot take because of a specific medication allergy.

Other Less Common Causes

Latex
Although once on the rise due to latex gloves increasingly being used to protect against infection, the number of people having anaphylaxis from latex is now decreasing because of increased awareness of the problem and as a result, decreased exposure. Non-latex alternatives for gloves and other medical supplies that were once made of latex are now commonplace. There are 2 types of latex allergy. The more common type is contact, also called *delayed-type allergy,* which comes on gradually and usually causes skin symptoms on the hands. It is a nuisance but not a disabling problem. The second, *immediate-type allergy,* is more serious and can result in anaphylaxis.

Symptoms of immediate-type allergy may occur when an allergic person touches latex, breathes in tiny particles, or is exposed to latex during surgery, dental work, or contact with other medical personnel who use latex gloves. Be sure to warn your child's dentist if your child has been diagnosed as having immediate-type latex allergy.

Exercise
Exercise can be a rare cause of anaphylaxis in children; it is more common in adults. In some rare cases, the child needs to have eaten a certain food just before or just after the period of vigorous exercise. This type of reaction is called *food-associated exercise-induced anaphylaxis.*

Idiopathic or Unknown Causes
In some cases a cause is never identified despite hard searching by the pediatrician. This type of reaction is called *idiopathic anaphylaxis,* meaning the cause of the anaphylaxis is unknown.

Chapter 7

Allergy Treatments

*I*n the best-case scenario, the ideal treatment for allergies is to avoid the substances that trigger symptoms. Of course, this is often impossible because many allergens are always in the air around us. Fortunately we now have an array of effective medications that help control symptoms. If medications don't do the trick, allergy shots (immunotherapy) are another solution.

Marissa and her parents are thrilled at the improvement in the teenager's overall well-being. About 9 months ago, their pediatrician referred Marissa to an allergy specialist who diagnosed her as having chronic allergic rhinitis or hay fever. Many people have hay fever in the spring and summer when pollen is heavy, but Marissa has the typical symptoms of runny, itchy nose; itchy eyes; and sneezing all year-round. In addition, her hay fever symptoms were worsened by frequent sinus infections. The results of skin tests confirmed that the teenager was allergic to many substances found outdoors and indoors, including dust mites, cat dander, mold, and grass pollen.

The allergy specialist put Marissa on a three-pronged treatment plan. The allergist recommended several measures to control dust mites in her bedroom, advised against using a humidifier in the house, and asked that the family cat be kept entirely outdoors. In addition, the physician instructed Marissa to use a cortisone-type nasal spray and take an antihistamine tablet every morning. The allergist also prescribed a decongestant nasal spray for Marissa to use only when she felt sinus congestion or an infection developing. In the hope of being able to control her allergies with fewer medications over time, Marissa decided to start immunotherapy (allergy shots) and has faithfully kept to the schedule for 8 months.

Now everything seems to be falling into place. Marissa's nose symptoms are much less severe—she doesn't need to stay near a tissue box; she is sleeping better; and she feels she has more energy. What's more, Marissa hasn't had a single sinus infection since starting the treatment program.

*P*hysicians employ a 3-point strategy to control allergies.

1. Avoidance to reduce allergen exposure
2. Medications to control and prevent symptoms
3. Allergen-specific immunotherapy (allergy shots), where appropriate, to decrease children's sensitivity

Allergen Avoidance to Reduce Exposure

Allergen avoidance begins at home for 2 important reasons. First, home is where it's easiest to control exposures. And second, indoor allergens found in our homes (see "Common Allergens on the Home Front" on the next page) are often the main causes of symptoms. That's because they are often present at fairly high levels even when a home is regularly cleaned. Moreover, children are exposed to them repeatedly and for long periods because home is where children spend most of their time. Measures to reduce allergen exposure may take some planning and effort, but they are a very effective way to prevent allergy symptoms.

Dust Mite Control

When you know that dust mites (see "Dust Mites to Dust" on page 62) are among the causes of your child's allergic symptoms, you may want to reach for the vacuum cleaner every time you spy a trace of dust on the furniture. But vacuuming may not be the solution. Use of a normally efficient vacuum cleaner stirs up clouds of fine dust that can hang about in the air for up to 8 hours and make sneezing, runny nose, and itchiness worse. It's best to wait until your allergic child is out of the house—at school for the day, for example—before vacuuming. Or to avoid stirring up dust, invest in a vacuum cleaner with a high-efficiency particulate air (HEPA) filter. To keep household dust levels down, clean all non-carpeted floors at least once a week with a damp mop and use a damp cloth to wipe flat surfaces, louver blinds, window ledges, and picture frames.

Air-conditioning and keeping doors and windows closed are effective ways to keep your home free of allergens and irritants brought in by air from the outside. While it may be too costly to install air-conditioning throughout your home, you may find an economical way to install a unit in your allergic child's bedroom. This could help him sleep better at night and provide a low-allergen retreat on days when the pollen count is high. Air-conditioner filters should be checked and cleaned regularly, and sprayed with an anti-mildew aerosol to control the growth of molds.

Common Allergens on the Home Front

- Dust (contains dust mites and finely ground particles from other allergens such as cockroaches, pollen, mold, and animal dander)
- Furry animals (cats, dogs, guinea pigs, gerbils, rabbits, and other pets)
- Pollen (trees, grasses, and weeds)
- Fungi (includes molds too small to be seen with the naked eye)
- Clothing and toys made, trimmed, or stuffed with animal hair

Less Common Allergens

- Latex (household articles such as rubber gloves, toys, balloons; elastic in socks, underwear, and other clothing; airborne particles)
- Seed dusts (beanbag toys and cushions)
- Bacterial enzymes (used to manufacture enzyme bleaches and cleaning products)
- Airborne dust from grain elevators, barns, and haylofts (in rural areas)

Families may find their allergic members have fewer symptoms when room air is filtered through a HEPA air cleaner. However, air filtration should complement, not replace, measures to control mites. In fact, air cleaners do not significantly reduce mite exposure and should not be recommended for dust mite control. A HEPA air cleaner can be installed centrally in a forced-air ventilation system, or used as a portable room unit and left on at night in your child's bedroom (see below). When you run a room HEPA cleaning unit, make sure the windows of the room are shut and the bedroom door is closed.

Your Allergic Child's Bedroom

Because your allergic child spends more time in the bedroom than in any other single location, it's a good idea to begin allergen control there. But if your child is highly allergic or several members of the family suffer from allergy symptoms, you may decide to extend many of the suggestions for allergen control from the bedroom throughout the rest of the house. Modifications suggested for the bedroom generally apply to other rooms as well.

Dust Mites to Dust

Dust mites are the main source of allergens in house dust. It's difficult for many people who are allergic to accept that these creatures, invisible except under a microscope, can be present in large numbers even in a thoroughly cleaned home. Some are convinced only when symptoms improve as a result of mite-containment measures.

Dust mites are members of the same family as spiders. Too small to be seen with the naked eye, they find a home wherever humans live. Dust mites don't ask for much in life. They feed on any protein that comes their way and find easy pickings in the dead skin scales that humans shed every day. Apart from this simple diet, they need only a moderately warm, moist atmosphere, with a temperature of 65°F or higher and humidity around 65%. Bedding is the ideal dust mite home; after all, bedding offers warmth, sufficient moisture, plenty of skin, and fibrous materials to which dust mites can cling with their barbed legs. They also thrive in upholstered furniture, clothing, soft toys, and carpets.

The dust mite eats and excretes pellets of feces that are about the size of pollen grains, and finds other dust mites, with which it produces many offspring. Their fecal pellets enter the general household dust to become the main source of allergens. Eventually, as mites die off, their dried-out carcasses, composed of allergenic proteins, also join the dust. Over years, they can add many pounds to the weight of a mattress.

The watchword for allergen control should be, "Simplify!" Throughout your home, get rid of dust catchers and put out-of-season clothing and articles that are used only occasionally into accessible storage. Use bedroom storage only for clothing and objects in current use.

Canopy beds and bunk beds are not good choices for allergic youngsters. The drapes on canopy beds are dust catchers, and bunk beds release an invisible shower of dust and mites over the lower bunk every time the child in the top bunk stirs in his sleep.

All beds in the bedroom should be treated identically, including spare beds that are only occasionally used. Mattresses, box springs, and pillows should be encased in impermeable dust-proof zippered casings. Seal zippers all along their length with duct tape to prevent leakage of dust mites and other allergens. Casings for bedding are available through catalogs, specialized retailers, and bedding departments of some major retailers (see Appendix C). A water bed may be better than a regular bed for a child who is allergic to dust mites. However, some water beds are unsuitable because they have quilting or padding that can harbor dust mites. Vacuuming is not an efficient way to remove live mites from carpeting and bedding. However, once dead, the mites cling less to their fibrous homes and are somewhat easier to vacuum up.

Applied periodically, benzyl benzoate foam or powder and other allergy products obtainable through catalogs and specialized retailers may lower levels of mite allergens in carpets and upholstered furniture. Follow the safety directions on containers to reduce your family's exposure to the chemicals. Benzyl benzoate, for example, should not be inhaled by anyone of any age, nor should it come in contact with the skin. To be safe, children should not be in the house while it is being applied and until after it is vacuumed up.

Keep Humidity Low to Discourage Mites

Dust mites flourish when the humidity is around 75% to 80%. These tiny cousins of spiders need water to survive but have no means of conserving it in their tissues. When the surrounding humidity falls below 50%, mites soon shrivel up and die. Thus, reducing household humidity can drastically reduce the dust mite population. A dehumidifier is useful for drying out the air. Take care to empty the water pan daily and scour it to stop the growth of microscopic molds (see page 66).

Avoid pillows, comforters, and cushions stuffed with down, feathers, or kapok. Replace woolen blankets with washable synthetics. Use only pillows and comforters stuffed with synthetic fibers and replace pillows every 2 to 3 years. Your child should take his own pillow on sleepovers and when traveling.

Use only synthetic or easily washable, lightweight, natural fiber fabrics to furnish your child's room. Mites and molds multiply in natural materials such as wool. Fabrics should be flat-weave (eg, percale, chintz), not napped (eg, chenille, velour). Sheets and pillowcases should be washed weekly; all other bedding, every 2 or 3 weeks. Dust mites can survive a lengthy wash in warm, soapy water. Wash all bedding for no less than 10 minutes on the hot water cycle (not warm), then place it in the dryer at the highest setting to kill any remaining dust mites. Although many people prefer the feel and smell of laundry fresh from the clothesline, laundry dried outdoors can worsen allergies because pollens and other airborne allergens may collect on the clothes and bedding.

Humidifier Use Can Promote Growth of Mites and Molds

Any increase in humidity, such as when a humidifier is used, will encourage mites and molds to grow in your child's room. If your child has problems with croup or other breathing difficulties, ask your pediatrician's advice about the best way to ensure that the air in the bedroom is moist enough to breathe comfortably but dry enough to discourage mites and molds.

Check your child's toy box periodically and get rid of toys that are no longer wanted or being used. Sweep the toy box and air it out from time to time to get rid of dust and prevent mold growth. Wash plastic toys periodically in soapy water or put them through a cycle in the dishwasher, if you have one. If your child can't be parted from a favorite soft toy, wash it regularly in hot water with bedding, or seal it in a plastic bag and leave it in the freezer overnight once a week to kill dust mites.

Unframed maps, posters, and prints can be used to brighten up walls, but fabric pennants and hangings, three-dimensional sculptural decorations, and picture frames catch dust and are best kept for another part of the house or relegated to storage. Sadly, books harbor molds and bookshelves gather dust. Store books in another room (dust them regularly) and try to keep only the current issues of newspapers, magazines, and comics.

Houseplants should be kept out of your child's room. Some allergy specialists advise getting rid of potted plants in all areas of the house because plants, particularly their soil, can be a source of mold. If you cultivate houseplants, wipe the leaves regularly with water for the plants' sake and to keep dust away from your allergic child.

Mildew-resistant paint is a better choice for bedroom walls than wallpaper. Molds can grow on the paper and in the adhesive paste.

To keep out pollen and environmental contaminants, your child's bedroom windows should be left closed as much as possible. Lightweight, washable curtains or vertical vinyl shades are suitable window coverings. Curtains should be washed at least once a month and vinyl shades dusted weekly with a damp sponge or dust-retentive tack cloth. Shutters, venetian and other horizontal blinds, drapes, and elaborate valances are not the best choice for your allergic child's bedroom; they are dust traps that may make allergy symptoms worse.

Bare wood, tile, and vinyl or linoleum are best for bedroom floors, rather than wall-to-wall carpeting. If a small amount of rug is desired, choose flat-weave or low-pile area and accent rugs made of cotton or synthetic fiber in small sizes that make it easy to wash and dry them frequently.

Odors, even pleasant smelling, can cause problems for allergic children. Avoid using potpourri, incense, and solid, wick, or spray room deodorizers. Potpourri can harbor molds and may contain spices and other irritating or allergenic particles that enter the air. The smell from room deodorizers can irritate sensitive mucous membranes in the nose of an allergic child or irritate the airways of a child with asthma.

Heating Systems

Dust and molds may collect in heating ducts and fill the air when a forced-air–type furnace is in operation. Baseboard heating and radiant heat are preferable to forced-air systems in homes in which people have allergies. Unfortunately, the cost of replacing a heating system is more than most families can manage. Where possible, the best solution is to seal off the heating vents in your child's bedroom with aluminum covers and tape to prevent dust-laden air from entering. Use other ways, if possible, to keep the child warm at night (eg, superwarm pajamas). Ask your heating company to replace the standard fiberglass furnace filters with more efficient filters that are better traps for dust and allergens.

Animal Allergies

Cats and dogs are among the most frequent causes of allergies. If your child is sensitive to other allergens, it is likely that with a pet—especially an indoor pet—in the home, she will also develop an animal allergy sooner or later.

When family history makes it likely that a baby or young child will develop allergies, it's best to postpone adopting a pet for several years until you are certain that your child is not allergic. In the case of an animal that has been part of the family since before the arrival of a child with allergies, decisions can be more difficult, especially when older children have formed strong attachments to the pet. It should be noted, though, that some research has begun to make allergy specialists confused about what to recommend for pet ownership. There are some interesting studies of children growing up with pet animals in the house that suggest exposure to 2 or more dogs or cats from birth (not later) may in fact decrease the later development of allergies and asthma.

Maybe It's OK to Keep Fido

Results of some recent research are laying waste to the common opinion that pets and children prone to allergies don't mix.

Studies that followed hundreds of children from birth to the school-aged years compared those exposed during infancy to cats or dogs with those who were not exposed to these animals. Results were the opposite of what the investigators expected—children exposed to 2 or more indoor pets early on were almost half as likely to develop common allergies to not only dogs and cats, but also to dust mites, grass, ragweed, and mold.

Researchers believe that children living with these animals are probably exposed to higher levels of something called *endotoxins*. Endotoxins are natural compounds secreted from bacteria that are commonly found in the intestines and feces of all animals, including cats and dogs. Exposure to endotoxins is thought to force the body's immune system to develop a different pattern of response that makes one less likely to become allergic.

But beware—this protective effect against developing allergies is not 100%. Plenty of kids will still go on to have allergies to their environment, including the family pet, so until researchers understand more about all of this, it is too early to recommend families run out and get animals to protect their child from developing hay fever and asthma. You are bound to be the one where the protection did not occur and left with having to sadly get rid of Fido or Puss and Boots for the sake of your allergic child.

When severe pet allergies are established, the kindest course is to find a new home for the animal. However, if you can't part with your pet, provide shelter and restraints to let it live outside. If this is not a practical solution, groom and bathe the animal frequently to reduce shedding of allergenic particles and hair, and keep it strictly out of your allergic child's bedroom and play areas. Mattress covers, air cleaners, and carpet removal are also useful to reduce exposure to animal allergens. When considering a pet, look into the possibility of an unusual but easily maintained animal. For example, allergic children do not have problems with fish or reptiles in a terrarium.

Give teachers and school personnel full information about your child's animal allergies. A highly allergic child may develop symptoms if animals (typically rabbits, birds, or small rodents) live in the classroom or come to school on visits. Made aware of the severity of your child's symptoms, teachers may reconsider the type of classroom animal (perhaps turtles or lizards instead of gerbils) and make sure that animals brought on special visits stay in another part of the building.

Pollens

Plants and trees that cause allergy problems have wind-borne pollen that is typically produced in clusters of small, nondescript flowers. By contrast, plants that rely on insects rather than wind for pollination generally have larger, bright, fragrant flowers with larger, sticky pollen grains that are not dispersed in the air. These plants are typically nonallergenic. In general, the prettier the plant, the less likely it is to be allergenic. Children with allergies to insect venom should keep away from bright flowers that attract bees (see also Chapter 6).

Pollen counts rise and lead to symptoms when the weather is dry, warm, and breezy. But people with hay fever and asthma may also find that their symptoms worsen during thunderstorms, when atmospheric conditions help to break down pollen grains, releasing allergen-bearing granules. No matter how high or low the pollen count, daily outdoor pollen levels are highest, on average, in the morning. It's a good idea to concentrate on indoor activities during pollen season, especially if you can keep the windows shut and the air conditioner running.

Molds and Fungi

Spores from molds and fungi get less attention than pollens, although they may be a very important cause of allergies. When air samples are measured for pollen and spore counts, spores are usually much more numerous than pollen grains. Spores are in the air all year long. Damp, mild weather promotes mold and fungus growth; warm, breezy weather favors circulation of spores on air currents. A mold-allergic youngster has a good excuse for avoiding outdoor chores that stir up molds in decomposing plant material, such as raking lawn clippings and fallen leaves.

While molds are everywhere outdoors, they can also be found indoors, especially where the humidity is above 40%. Molds thrive on organic materials such as wood, cotton and other natural fibers, wicker, straw, paper, and leather. *Mildew,* another name for mold, is almost always a problem in bathrooms. House plants that are watered often can harbor mold in their soil and on the plant itself. Molds are highly opportunistic, and given the right amount of moisture in the air, can gain a foothold even on synthetic surfaces that offer no other source of nutrition.

To discourage molds and fungi, clean household surfaces regularly with an ammonia-based cleaner, diluted household bleach, or a fungicidal spray and keep indoor humidity below 40%. Shy away from using humidifiers. Any area of your home that has been damaged by water can harbor mold; if there are leaks (eg, in the roof), find and seal them.

Medications to Suppress Symptoms

Several effective, easy-to-use medications are available to treat allergy symptoms. Some are available by prescription; others, over the counter. As with any medications, over-the-counter products should be used only with the advice of your child's pediatrician.

Antihistamines

Antihistamines, the longest-established allergy medications, dampen the allergic reaction mainly by suppressing the effects of histamine (itching, swelling, and mucus production) in the tissues. For mild allergy symptoms, your pediatrician may recommend one of the anti-histamines widely available over the counter. Children who don't like to swallow tablets may prefer the medication in syrup, chewable, or melt-away form. Some over-the-counter anti-histamines, in particular the "old-generation" type, have drowsiness as a possible side effect. For this reason, it's best to give the dose in the evening, which can relieve symptoms and help your child with allergies sleep better. However, there are "new-generation" antihista-mines that do not cause drowsiness; some need a prescription, while others are available over the counter. Ask your pediatrician whether these non-sedating antihistamines are appropriate for your child.

Antihistamines can be useful for controlling the itchiness that accompanies hay fever, ecze-ma, and hives. Your pediatrician may advise your child to take them regularly or just as needed. However, in general, antihistamines work best when taken every day rather than intermittently. New-generation antihistamines have the convenience of once-a-day dosing, which makes it easy for children to use them daily. Antihistamine nasal sprays are also avail-able for hay fever. They work locally in the nose to reduce symptoms. Some kids shy away from nose sprays and prefer using the antihistamines taken by mouth.

Decongestants

For hay fever sufferers, antihistamines help stop runny nose, itching, and sneezing, but they have little effect on nasal congestion or stuffiness. To cover the range of symptoms, an antihistamine is often given together with a decongestant, sometimes combined in a single medication. In contrast to older antihistamines, which tend to make people sleepy, decongestants taken by mouth can cause stimulation. Children taking these medications may act hyper, feel anxious, have a racing heart, or find it difficult to get to sleep. Because of these possible side effects, it is best to avoid using long-term daily decongestants to control your child's nasal congestion, and instead, use another type of medication, such as a nasal corticosteroid spray (see below).

Decongestant treatment can be given topically with nose drops or sprays, but these medications have to be used carefully, and only for a short while, because prolonged use can lead to a rebound effect. The resulting stuffy nose is more difficult to treat than the original allergy symptoms.

Cromolyn

Cromolyn sodium is sometimes recommended to prevent nasal allergy symptoms. This medication can be used every day for chronic problems or just for a limited period when a child is likely to encounter allergens. The medication is available without prescription as a nasal spray; it is taken 3 or 4 times a day. Nasal cromolyn has almost no side effects, but it's potency is not high, and because it requires frequent administration, it is hard to use on a regular basis in a consistent way.

Corticosteroids

Corticosteroids, a category of medications also called steroids or cortisones, are highly effective for allergy treatment and are widely used to stop symptoms. They are available as creams (ointments), nasal sprays, asthma inhalers, and pills or liquids. Steroid creams are a mainstay of treatment for children with eczema. As long as they are used sparingly, at the lowest strength that does the job, steroid creams are very safe and effective. They control the rash when applied twice a day, or even once a day if the rash is not severe. Nasal sprays that contain a compound derived from cortisone have become the most effective form of treatment for patients with nasal allergy problems. Once-daily dosing is usually enough. These medications work best if used on a regular daily schedule, rather than with as-needed, interrupted dosing. No problems have emerged so far over many years in patients using cortisone nasal sprays over the long term. Corticosteroid asthma inhalers are frequently used for treatment of asthma; like steroid nasal sprays, they are highly effective in controlling symptoms (see also Chapter 11).

Steroid pills or liquid are sometimes used for short periods to bring allergy or asthma symptoms under control so that other measures can have a chance to work. In rare cases, a child may have to take oral steroids every day or on alternate days to control severe allergy problems. Steroid pills and liquid should be used sparingly because they carry a higher risk of side effects, including weight gain, high blood pressure, cataracts, and slowing of growth.

Allergy Immunotherapy

Immunotherapy, or allergy shots, may be recommended to reduce your child's sensitivity to airborne allergens. This form of treatment consists of giving a person material he is allergic to, by injection, with the goal of changing his immune system and making him less allergic to that material. Not every allergy problem can or needs to be treated with allergy shots, but treatment of respiratory allergies to pollen, dust mites, and outdoor molds is often successful. Immunotherapy for cat (and possibly dog) allergy can also be very effective, but allergy specialists advise that avoidance is the best way to manage animal allergies in children. Immunotherapy takes some time to work and demands patience and commitment. The treatment is given by injecting gradually stronger doses of allergen extract once or twice a week at first, then at longer intervals—for example, once every 2 weeks, then every 3 weeks, and eventually every 4 weeks. The effect of the extract reaches its maximum after 6 to 12 months of injections.

Surgery and Allergy Treatment

Surgery is not a treatment for allergies, but surgery is sometimes performed to correct a condition that is contributing to severe upper respiratory symptoms. For example, the removal of enlarged adenoid tissue (known as an *adenoidectomy*) from the upper throat, just behind the nose, can eliminate an obstruction, thereby increasing airflow through the nose. Adenoidectomy is also sometimes done to eliminate a possible contributing factor in recurrent sinusitis (see Chapter 4, page 34). In some cases, a minor surgical procedure is done to drain pus that is backed up in the sinuses.

Adults sometimes have a crooked (deviated) nasal septum, the wall of cartilage that separates the 2 nasal cavities. A deviated septum can make it difficult to breathe through the nose. Fortunately, this is very uncommon in children; therefore, surgery to correct a deviation is rarely, if ever, needed.

After a number of months of immunotherapy, the youngster usually feels his allergy symptoms are better. Allergy injections are often continued for 3 to 5 years, and then a decision is made whether to stop them. Many children do fine after the shots are stopped and have little or no return of their symptoms.

Complementary Allergy Therapies

Your child's allergy treatment should start with your pediatrician, who may refer you to a pediatric allergy specialist for additional evaluations and treatments. Some parents also seek relief through alternative or complementary therapies. Many such therapies are based on traditional remedies that have not been proven effective by scientific testing. Several complementary approaches (eg, acupuncture, acupressure) have been promoted as alternatives to help alleviate symptoms, but it is unlikely that any could produce natural immunity to allergies, as immunotherapy does. If you are thinking about trying an alternative therapy, be sure to talk with your child's treating physician beforehand to avoid the risk of interactions between conventional and alternative therapies.

Herbal extracts should never be used unless you first check with your child's doctor because some may be chemically related to your child's allergens and thus capable of causing or worsening symptoms. A compress soaked in camomile tea may soothe the inflammation and itching of hives but can produce an allergic reaction in a person sensitive to plants in the aster family. The sticky, clear gel (not the yellow juice) from inside aloe leaves may also soothe the skin. Witch hazel is often promoted to relieve skin troubles; however, it is effective only if it is brewed from dried bark, leaves, and stems that contain *tannins*—plant chemicals that tighten and soothe the skin. The steam-distilled witch hazel extracts sold in pharmacies do not contain tannins. Congestion of the nose and sinuses may be eased by breathing steam from water in which cloves, bayberry, or eucalyptus leaves have been boiled. Interestingly, cromolyn (see page 68 and Chapter 11) is extracted from a plant traditionally used by Mediterranean folk healers to ease breathing problems.

Advice from a registered dietitian may help you to plan meals and find alternative sources for important nutrients when your child is allergic to primary foods (eg, milk, wheat). However, steer clear of self-styled "nutritionists" who use methods such as hair analysis or morning saliva samples to evaluate your child's allergies and general health. Time and again, these "healers" prove to have no scientific training in diet and health. Instead, they often have ties to producers of vitamin and mineral supplements. They are interested in marketing superfluous products, not in promoting health through good nutrition. If your child has nutritional issues related to food allergies, ask your pediatrician to refer you to a qualified dietitian with experience in pediatric allergies.

PART 3
LIVING WITH ASTHMA

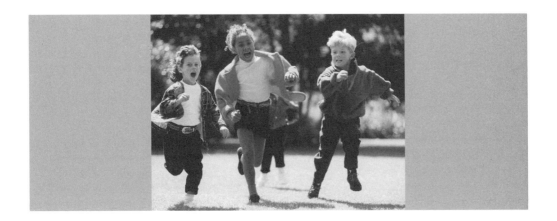

Chapter 8

Asthma Overview

*O*ne of the surprising facts about asthma is that it is such a common disease. More than 23 million Americans have the condition and more than one-quarter of them are children younger than 18 years. The rates are steadily rising, though no one can state exactly why. There are probably many reasons for the increase. Not only are we learning more about what causes asthma, but we also have more accurate methods of diagnosing the disorder and better ways to treat it, even in very young children.

Andrew, who just turned 3, sees his pediatrician for his third bout of bronchitis this winter. To Andrew's mother it seems that every time he catches a cold, it "moves into his chest." With each episode he coughs a lot and for a long time, and this time his mother noticed wheezing as well. Their pediatrician confirms the wheezing during the examination. Andrew's mother tells the doctor that after the last bout of bronchitis, Andrew never seemed to get entirely back to normal. He tends to cough when running about, as well as in the middle of the night. Andrew is losing sleep and missing a lot of preschool because of frequent respiratory illnesses. This, in turn, means that his mother is missing work because she has to stay home to take care of him.

When the pediatrician brings up the possibility that Andrew might have asthma, his mother is relieved and concerned—relieved because the diagnosis would help explain his illnesses, but concerned because asthma is a serious condition. Her brother Tim had asthma when he was young, and she remembers how their mother had to stay with Tim when he was in the hospital.

The pediatrician reassures the family that Andrew's asthma is not severe and that asthma can be managed easily with proper treatment. He recommends a regular medication program to control Andrew's airway inflammation.

When Andrew's mother calls her brother to relay the news, she is surprised to learn that although his asthma is much better overall than when he was a child, Tim still develops asthma symptoms when he catches a cold or jogs. It turns out that Andrew and Tim are taking some of the same asthma medications.

At the follow-up visit a few weeks later, Andrew's cough and chest symptoms are much better, thanks to the asthma medication program. He is back to playing outside without coughing and is sleeping through the night.

. . . .

*A*sthma may appear at any age; however, between 80% and 90% of children with asthma develop symptoms by age 4 or 5 years. Fortunately, in the vast majority of cases, symptoms are mild to moderately severe. When the condition is properly managed with medications and environmental measures, most severe, potentially incapacitating flare-ups can be prevented. There are often early warning signs that a child is at risk for developing asthma—eczema starting in the early months, frequent lower respiratory symptoms and problems appearing before the first birthday, and having a family history of asthma.

Asthma Among Minority Groups

Asthma is a serious and growing problem among minority groups. About 9 or 10 out of every 100 African American children have asthma, compared with a rate of 7 or 8 out of 100 for white US children. African Americans also tend to require hospital admission more often and have more severe and potentially fatal asthma attacks. In part, the rate may be higher because African Americans who have asthma are more likely to live in the inner city where there are higher concentrations of asthma triggers such as air pollution and dust that contains debris from household pests like cockroaches.

Among American children and adolescents aged 18 years and younger, the rate of asthma increased by more than 70% between 1982 and 1994, but this increase seems to be leveling off somewhat except for those children younger than 5 years. Although part of the increase may be because of better methods of identifying people with asthma, the rise is real and disturbing.

Researchers are working to find links between the increase in asthma and environmental problems. Air pollution may be one contributing factor; more than 60% of Americans with asthma live in areas that don't meet federal air quality standards. However, blaming the environment and air pollution is not entirely fair and oversimplifies the problem because the overall quality of the air we breathe is actually better today than 40 years ago, when the first Clean Air Act was passed.

Smoking is another contributing factor. One American Lung Association study found that children's wheezing attacks could be reduced by 20% if parents didn't smoke at home.

The General Has Spoken

Passive smoking is the inhalation of smoke, called *secondhand smoke* or *environmental tobacco smoke,* from tobacco products used by others. It occurs when tobacco smoke permeates any environment, causing its inhalation by people within that environment, such as kids. Toxins linger in the air and in fabrics long after a smoker leaves the room. Secondhand smoke as a result of a parent or other family member smoking in the house of a child with asthma can be an important and potent trigger for asthma flare-ups and the reason for overall poor control of the child's asthma.

The 2006 US Surgeon General report on smoking revealed some additional scary facts about passive smoking.

- Many millions of Americans, children and adults, are exposed to secondhand smoke in their homes and workplaces despite substantial progress in tobacco control.

- Secondhand smoke exposure causes disease and premature death in children and adults who do not smoke.

- Children exposed to secondhand smoke are at an increased risk for sudden infant death syndrome (SIDS), acute respiratory infections, ear problems, and more severe asthma. Smoking by parents causes respiratory symptoms and slows lung growth in their children.

- The scientific evidence shows that there is no safe level of exposure to secondhand smoke.

Steps to Reduce Exposure

- Do not smoke while you are pregnant.

- Make your home a smoke-free zone. Remove ashtrays from your home and place signs in your home asking people not to smoke.

- Protect your children. Let caregivers and babysitters know that you do not allow smoking in your home or around your children.

- Support those who decide to quit smoking.

- Do not allow smoking in your car.

- Patronize smoke-free restaurants. Do not let your teens work in restaurants or workplaces where smoking is permitted.

- Do not allow people to smoke in any location where children spend time.

Some researchers have noted that people today have fewer infections, thanks to improved standards of cleanliness, hygiene, and overall public health. They believe these improvements cause the immune system to switch from fighting infections to producing allergy antibodies. This has been labeled the "too clean" theory or "hygiene hypothesis" (see "The 'Too Clean' Theory or the 'Hygiene Hypothesis'" in Chapter 4 on page 32). This hypothesis could explain the higher rate of asthma being seen since allergies and asthma are often linked in childhood.

A sedentary lifestyle—hours spent in front of the TV or computer rather than in active pastimes—leads to obesity, and children who are overweight have a higher rate of asthma, not to mention an increased risk of other diseases in adulthood. Children who spend long periods indoors are exposed for longer periods to the full range of indoor allergens, including dust mites and pet dander, as well as secondhand smoke and irritating fumes and odors.

Researchers agree that adults and children alike need to identify and avoid substances that trigger their asthma attacks, whether those substances are environmental pollutants or individual allergens. They agree, too, that most fatal asthma attacks occur because the disease is poorly controlled on a day-to-day basis. At highest risk for serious asthma attacks are those who don't seek regular medical care and instead resort to emergency departments only after they develop severe breathing difficulties. About 4,500 people die from asthma each year in the United States. Many of these deaths are the result of inadequate general asthma care and occur because treatment is delayed, often because the physician or patient underestimated the severity of the attack.

The sad and ironic aspect about these asthma deaths is that the outlook for children with asthma has never been better. A number of developments over the last decade or so have led to substantial improvements in asthma care (see chapters 11 and 13). We have better tools for diagnosing asthma than ever before. And thanks to a better understanding of the causes of asthma, medications have been developed that are more effective because they are targeted to the specific mechanisms behind the symptoms (see Chapter 11). They also have fewer side effects than older medications.

As we have developed better ways to diagnose and manage asthma, there has been a dramatic shift in attitudes toward the disease. While nobody should ignore the fact that asthma is a chronic, serious condition, children with asthma are no longer restricted, as many once were, to a life of being indoors or on the sidelines. Children with asthma are now encouraged to take part in any sport or activity, no matter how demanding, that is appropriate for their age and development.

How the Lungs Work

To understand what's going on in asthma, you have to know how the lungs and airways function in normal conditions. The respiratory system is often pictured as an upside-down, hollowed-out tree. The trunk is the *trachea,* or windpipe, a wide, fairly stiff tube that links the nose and throat to the lungs. The base of the trachea branches off into 2 large tubes (mainstem bronchi), each of which leads to a lung. Once in the lung, each bronchus splits into several smaller bronchial tubes, and each of these branches into smaller tubes called *bronchioles.* Each bronchiole, in turn, branches into many pockets filled with thousands of tiny air sacs called *alveoli.* Bronchial tubes have a wall ringed with muscle on the outside and an inner lining layer that produces mucus that coats the inside of the tubes.

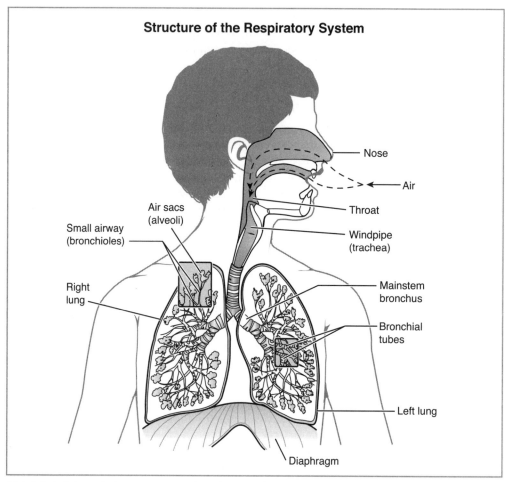

Structure of the Respiratory System

- Nose
- Air
- Throat
- Windpipe (trachea)
- Air sacs (alveoli)
- Small airway (bronchioles)
- Right lung
- Mainstem bronchus
- Bronchial tubes
- Left lung
- Diaphragm

Air is inhaled through the nose or mouth, and passes through the larynx (voice box) into the windpipe, or trachea (a muscular tube). The trachea branches into a large pipe, the mainstem bronchus, leading into each lung. Each mainstem bronchus then branches into several bronchial tubes, which have an outer wall ringed with muscle and a lining that produces a mucus coating. The bronchial tubes split into several smaller tubes, each of which branches into even smaller tubes called bronchioles. In turn, the bronchioles branch into pockets filled with thousands of tiny air sacs called alveoli.

When we breathe in through the nose or mouth, air passes into the trachea and down through the progressively smaller airways to the alveoli, where the actual process of respiration takes place (there are about 300 million little air sacs in every pair of lungs). There, oxygen extracted from the air passes into the bloodstream and on to all the other tissues. To complete the exchange, waste gases (carbon dioxide) pass out of the blood and back into the alveoli, where they mix with leftover air and are exhaled from the lungs.

What Happens in Asthma?

Asthma throws a wrench into the normally smooth-running airway. The airways of the typical child with asthma are inflamed, which makes them oversensitive, poised to react by narrowing whenever they come in contact with an asthma trigger. As a result, with asthma, airways become hyperresponsive or twitchy. They overreact with constriction and narrowing of the bronchial tubes when confronted with various materials and conditions to which people who don't have asthma have no reaction. For example, the lungs of any normal person in a building on fire with high levels of smoke are likely to react with constriction of the airways. This is a normal process believed to protect the lungs. By contrast, a child with asthma doesn't need the extreme conditions of a building on fire to develop airway constriction; he develops asthma symptoms when he is simply around one of his asthma triggers, catches a respiratory infection, or is exposed to an irritant such as a strong smell or tobacco smoke.

The tendency to become twitchy is probably present in the lungs from infancy, although in some cases symptoms may not emerge until much later. Researchers generally agree that asthma is a genetic condition; that is, it runs in families, along with nasal allergies, food allergies, and eczema, and can be inherited in the genes from either parent or both, although who inherits this condition is not entirely predictable. About 70% to 80% of children with asthma also have allergies (see Chapter 1), especially to airborne allergens such as pollen, dust mites, animal dander, and molds. Contact with an allergen (eg, cat dander) may set off an asthma attack, but it doesn't have to result in a full-blown attack for it to be a problem. New findings have shaken up and overturned many traditional views of asthma. For example, asthma was thought to occur in bouts, with quiet, symptom-free intervals in between. This is only partly true. The latest thinking is that the airways become persistently inflamed, swollen, and twitchy as a result of repeated exposures to asthma triggers, particularly those that cause allergies (allergens). The twitchy airways may not be inflamed enough to cause breathing problems, but it doesn't take much to push them into an acute attack. When an asthma trigger comes along, the person with inflamed airways begins to cough or wheeze or have chest tightness; if the reaction is severe, that person becomes short of breath or has a full-blown asthma attack.

Asthma Symptoms Are Often Worse at Night

Coughing and other symptoms that are usually worse at night are often a tip-off for asthma. Our lung function reaches its 24-hour low point in the early hours of the morning, and this reduction is even greater in people with asthma. Because of this, asthma often rears its ugly head more often in the nighttime. Emergency department visits for asthma are always higher late at night and into early morning hours.

In asthma, air passing through the bronchial tubes is blocked in 3 ways and to varying degrees. First, the muscular bands around the airways contract and squeeze the air passages tight. Next, white blood cells enter the tissues and release irritating chemicals that are produced by the immune system (see "What Happens During an Allergic Reaction" in Chapter 1 on page 5), causing inflammation and swelling in the lining of the airways and narrowing the passages. Finally, the bronchial mucous glands (we all have them, but they are more abundant in children with asthma) overproduce mucus, which further plugs the airways.

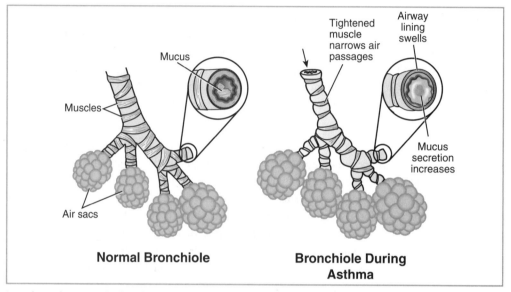

In asthma the muscular bands around the airways contract and squeeze the air passages tight. White blood cells enter the tissues and release irritating chemicals, causing inflammation, leading to swelling of the inner lining and further narrowing of the passages. Finally, mucous glands overproduce mucus, which aggravates the plugging up of the airways.

Recognizing Asthma

Many children suffer needlessly because those around them aren't aware of the warning signs of asthma and do not bring the signs to their pediatricians' attention. Asthma can masquerade for years as chronic or recurrent bronchitis, recurrent pneumonia, chronic cough, or lower respiratory infections. Discuss with your pediatrician the possibility that your child has asthma if he has these masquerading conditions. Also call your pediatrician for an appointment if your child

- Wheezes

- Coughs regularly, especially at night or with exertion

- Has a tight feeling in the chest

- Is often short of breath

Symptoms may not always be there; instead, they may occur occasionally, such as when your child plays energetically, laughs or cries, or sleeps. Perhaps you notice that your child wheezes or coughs when visiting a home in which someone smokes or has a cat. If symptoms come on at particular times, be sure to mention the circumstances to your pediatrician. The more facts your pediatrician has, the easier it is to diagnose asthma and the sooner treatment can start.

Mild, Moderate, Severe: What Do Grades Mean?

After confirming an asthma diagnosis, your pediatrician will grade the severity of your child's condition. This grading takes into account the frequency and severity of past and current asthma symptoms and the physical examination, and may include measures of lung function including spirometry or peak flow measurements. This information enables your pediatrician to select the right medication and determine the proper dose to keep the condition in check. (See "What Really Matters Is Control, Not Severity" below.) In making a decision about a child's asthma severity level, the first distinction to be made is whether your child has *intermittent* asthma (ie, just occasional problems) or *persistent* asthma (ie, more than occasional). Patients with persistent asthma can have mild, moderate, or severe asthma. Following are more details about the 4 asthma severity levels that arise by making this kind of distinction.

What Really Matters Is Control, Not Severity

It turns out that asthma severity categories are somewhat arbitrary and, in fact, were actually created more with adults in mind than children. They are just a general guide for the doctor seeing your child; your doctor realizes that asthma severity levels, particularly in children, can change over time, so reassessments need to take place on an ongoing basis to verify an individual child's present asthma severity. Furthermore, the 2007 National Heart, Lung, and Blood Institute "National Asthma Education and Prevention Program Expert Panel Report 3: Guidelines for the Diagnosis and Management of Asthma" make a strong point that the overall *control* of your child's asthma is really what is most important, not what the severity level happens to be at any time. Adjustments of treatment are based mainly on how well-controlled your child's asthma is when assessed at follow-up visits.

Intermittent Asthma

A child who has symptoms of wheezing and coughing no more than 2 days a week is considered to have intermittent asthma; nighttime flare-ups occur twice a month at most. Outside of these few episodes, a child with intermittent asthma is free of asthma symptoms.

Any child with asthma symptoms more often than 2 days a week or 2 nights per month, on average, is felt to no longer have intermittent asthma but *persistent* asthma. Persistent asthma has 3 levels of severity.

Mild Persistent Asthma

In *mild persistent* asthma, symptoms occur more than twice a week but less than once a day, and flare-ups may affect activity. Nighttime flare-ups occur more often than twice a month but less than once a week. Lung function is 80% of normal or greater.

Moderate Persistent Asthma

Asthma is classified as *moderate persistent* if symptoms occur daily. Flare-ups occur and usually last several days. Coughing and wheezing may disrupt the child's normal activities and make it difficult to sleep. Nighttime flare-ups may occur more than once a week. In moderate persistent asthma, lung function is roughly between 60% and 80% of normal, without treatment.

Severe Persistent Asthma

With *severe persistent* asthma, symptoms occur daily and often. They also frequently curtail the child's activities or disrupt his sleep. Lung function is less than 60% of the normal level without treatment. Severe is the least-common asthma level.

What Happens During an Asthma Attack?

As an attack happens, your child may begin coughing as she breathes. She then may feel chest tightness.

Soon she starts to wheeze, beginning with a slight whistling sound and continuing with a shrill rasp as she tries to get air into her lungs. She breathes fast, working so hard that you can see her abdomen going in and out, and her chest being sucked in on every breath. This effect is particularly noticeable in children, whose chests are small and flexible. The child may appear restless and fearful.

For a child who doesn't yet know how to get symptoms under control and live with asthma, even the thought of an asthma attack is frightening. She panics at the thought of feeling starved for air and struggling to breathe—an action the rest of us can perform without thinking about it.

Managing Asthma: Control Is Key

How you accept your child's asthma diagnosis may depend on whether you view life as a glass that's half empty or half full. For parents in the latter category, the knowledge comes as a relief. Finally, they can take the necessary steps to help their child live with asthma and lead a normal, active life. With avoidance of allergens and regular use of medications to calm airway inflammation, most attacks can be prevented. Additional medications can be held in reserve to cut off occasional flare-ups (see Chapter 11).

Recognizing that asthma can be a smoldering process going on in the airways all the time, doctors have changed the way they treat the condition. Now, instead of waiting until an attack occurs, their approach is to control the underlying silent inflammation with the aim of preventing flare-ups and severe breathing difficulties.

Daily control is the key. Children and their families can be taught to keep asthma symptoms under control, recognize warning signs, and head off serious attacks. Effective medications are available to quickly stop breathing difficulties. Modern medicines including handy inhalers make it easy to take medications to prevent wheezing with measured doses that go directly to the lungs, reducing the risk of side effects (see Chapter 11).

Severe, potentially fatal attacks occur most often in those whose asthma is not regularly monitored and controlled. Even though effective, convenient treatment is available, too many people still wait until their child's breathing becomes labored, then depend on a visit to a hospital emergency department to solve the problem. Unfortunately, by the time breathing difficulties have set in, it may be too late to stop a bad bout.

Most children with asthma have allergies, and many asthma attacks are set off by allergic reactions. Allergy skin or blood tests (see Chapter 2) can sometimes be important in your child's diagnostic evaluation for asthma. Once you know what substances he is allergic to, you can make special efforts to avoid them and thus help prevent many episodes.

Asthma Fables and Facts

Although our knowledge of asthma is expanding year by year, many people still cling to outdated beliefs about the disease. Following are some that are often repeated:

Asthma Fable	Asthma Fact
Asthma comes and goes.	Asthma is often an inflammatory condition that is always in the airways, even when the person is not having trouble breathing. Exposure to an asthma trigger can worsen symptoms, but the underlying condition never goes away, although it can be controlled with medications and environmental control measures.
Asthma is an emotional disorder; it's "all in the mind."	Asthma is a lung disease; it affects the airways, not the brain. It's true that symptoms may get worse when a person is under emotional stress, but this is probably more marked in adults and less so in children. Changes in the airways in asthma occur through physiological mechanisms, not emotional ones.
People with asthma should use medications only when they have attacks; otherwise, the medications lose their effect.	Regularly using medications is the only way to calm the underlying airway inflammation and prevent asthma flare-ups. Used at the correct dosage, daily medications do not lose their effect or cause uncomfortable side effects. Effective antiasthma medications include inhaled beta-agonists such as albuterol to stop attacks, and inhaled steroids, long-acting beta-agonists, and leukotriene modifiers to prevent attacks from occurring at all.

Asthma Fable	Asthma Fact
Asthma is just an annoying condition, not a real disease.	Asthma can kill when people do not get treatment to control the underlying condition and stop severe attacks. If everybody who needed medications used the proper ones to control symptoms and prevent flare-ups, hospitalizations and deaths from asthma would be greatly reduced.
Children grow out of asthma.	Most people who have asthma are born with a tendency to the condition and keep it for life. It is true many children get much better with age, and their asthma appears to go away completely. However, many have it return in adulthood. Other children who still have asthma are less likely to lose their asthma as they go in to their adult years.
Asthma clears up when you move to a warm, dry climate.	If the proper environmental measures are taken and medications are regularly used, people with asthma can live comfortably in any climate they prefer. Very rarely do people ever have to move out of a city or other area because of their asthma.

Chapter 9

Common Triggers and How to Identify Them

*A*sthma triggers are substances that start the chain of events leading to chronic *irritation and inflammation of the airways, and may eventually lead the inflamed airways into an acute asthma attack. To keep asthma in control, every youngster needs to identify his own personal triggers and learn to avoid them as much as possible.*

Six-year-old Beth has just been diagnosed as having asthma and allergic rhinitis (hay fever), and her pediatrician has put her on a regular medication program. Beth's parents wonder if her symptoms are related to the house they moved into a year before, her new school, the soccer fields where she often plays, or the cat they acquired after the family moved. Beth has had more problems with her asthma since starting soccer, but her mother can't tell whether the cause is the grass or the exercise. Although Beth never develops obvious asthma when around the cat, her mother notices that Beth's eyes itch and her nose is more runny in the mornings after the cat has slept in Beth's room. The house they had moved to is about 40 years old and has wall-to-wall carpeting. Beth's new school was built around the same time.

To clear up confusion, the family's pediatrician refers Beth to a pediatric allergist who performs allergy skin testing. Beth, afraid that the testing would hurt, is pleasantly surprised to find it isn't very painful. The test results show that Beth is allergic to dust mites, cat and dog dander, molds, and grass and tree pollen. The allergist explains that children like Beth, who have year-round asthma and allergic rhinitis, commonly have multiple allergies.

To help reduce Beth's exposure to allergy triggers, the family is asked to put the cat entirely outdoors and cancel plans to adopt a dog. The allergist advises Beth's parents on measures to control dust mites and molds in their home, with particular attention to minimizing these allergens in their daughter's bedroom. Fortunately, the house is air-conditioned, and the allergist recommends using the air-conditioning in spring and summer when pollen counts are high. Beth and her parents are relieved because they now know who the "enemy" is and—although they know it is hard to keep Beth completely from all of her triggers, especially the nonallergic ones like viral infections that flare up her asthma—they are ready to take action to improve Beth's breathing problems.

*O*ne minute your child is breathing normally as he plays, exercises, or sleeps. The next, he is wheezing, and in no time at all, he is struggling for breath and on his way to a full-blown asthma attack. By now, of course, you know that asthma doesn't appear out of the blue. First, your child's airways become inflamed and hyperalert as a result of sensitization. Then, when an asthma trigger comes along, like exposure to an allergen or a "cold," the state of alert erupts into an airway-system shutdown that make it difficult to breath.

> ### Common Asthma Triggers
>
> **Allergies**
> - Molds
> - Pollen
> - Dust mites
> - Cockroaches
> - Animals (especially cats and dogs)
>
> **Tobacco smoke**
>
> **Infections**
> - Viral respiratory infections, including colds
> - Sinus infections
>
> **Outdoor air pollution**
>
> **Indoor air pollution**
> - Aerosol sprays
> - Cooking fumes
> - Odors
> - Smoke (eg, wood fires, wood-burning stoves)

Not everybody with allergies has asthma, but the reverse is generally true, especially in children older than 4 years. Odds are that if your child has asthma, he also has hay fever (*allergic rhinitis;* see Chapter 4) and the allergens that bring on his hay fever are also often the triggers for his asthma. In your child's first year or two of life, he may have had the itchy, dry rash of eczema, possibly due to food sensitivity. Yet while 70% to 80% of children with asthma are allergic and allergens can inflame the airways, leading them to constrict, not all asthma triggers are allergens. Many nonallergenic substances can irritate the airway tree and prompt the body to respond by stepping up mucus production and tightening the bronchi. In this case, the body's reaction bypasses the immune system, which regulates all true allergic reactions (see Chapter 1). Examples of nonallergenic factors that can promote and trigger asthma include air pollution, emotional stress, cold air, exercise, and odors. But probably the most important and consistent nonallergenic-type triggers for asthma are viral respiratory infections and sinus infections. This is one of the reasons children with asthma have the toughest time getting through fall and winter seasons—that's when colds and viral infections appear on the scene. Whether it be from allergenic triggers, nonallergenic triggers, or both, repeated exposure can lead to chronic inflammation and acute and chronic asthma symptoms.

Symptoms Diary

Skin or blood tests can identify allergens that trigger your child's asthma. To help identify both types of triggers, your pediatrician may ask you to keep a symptoms diary for several weeks. You (and your child, if old enough) will use the diary to record the types of symptoms; when and where they occur (eg, when visiting Grandpa, who smokes cigars; during a sleepover at the home of a friend who has a cat); weather conditions at the time of the attack (eg, dry and breezy, humid and overcast, thunderstorm); how long symptoms last; what action is taken; and what happens to the symptoms after the action is taken. Information provided by the diary can help your pediatrician to focus on unusual or recurrent factors that should be further investigated.

Molds

Molds are all around us, indoors and out. They can flourish visibly or invisibly on almost any surface. Often they can be seen in the form of *mildew*—gray-black streaks and patches on the bathroom grout or refrigerator gaskets. Outdoors, they play a key role in the natural life cycle that breaks down vegetation into soil. Every time your child steps onto grass or soil, she sends a cloud of molds into the air. Mold spores float in the air, as pollen grains do. Most of them resettle on new sites, where they can proliferate to form new colonies, but some also enter the airways, where they can promote asthma in a susceptible person. Mold spore levels in the air are often higher than pollen levels, so they are common and important allergens. See Chapter 12 for suggestions on how to control molds and other asthma triggers.

It's impossible to get rid of outdoor molds, but you can help your child avoid the worst of them. While molds hang about in the air in almost any condition, windy weather is the worst for stirring up and circulating extra high levels of mold spores. Check your local newspaper for mold counts, which are usually reported along with pollen counts. Pollen and mold counts are also reported by local radio and TV stations and on the Internet. If possible, plan indoor activities and diversions for days when levels are high.

Pollens

Pollens are the microscopic granules produced and released by trees, grasses, and weeds. Different plants release pollen at different times, but the typical pollen season runs from early spring to late fall. The cycle begins with trees in the early spring, continues with grasses from late spring through the summer, and winds up with weed pollens in the fall. In some parts of the country where the climate is mild, pollination of all types occurs year-round.

Pollen counts indicate the number of pollen grains circulating in every cubic meter of air. Counts between 20 and 100 are levels that usually trigger symptoms in people with asthma and allergies; however, even at counts below 20, pollens can still be asthma triggers. As with molds, it's impossible to avoid pollens altogether. What's important is to take all possible measures to keep from needlessly exposing your child to these and other allergens (see Chapter 12).

Dust Mites, Cockroaches

In addition to acting as an irritating material, household dust may contain many different allergenic substances, including pollens, molds, dried-up insect bodies and feces, pet hair, and dander. Perhaps worst of all, dust contains dust mites and their feces (see Chapter 4, page 36), which are among the most common causes of allergies.

Skin or blood testing can show whether a child is allergic to dust mites; at least 25% of children with asthma have this sensitivity. These microscopic creatures have made their home with humans for so long that it's all but impossible to eradicate them from our dwellings, at least in temperate and warm climates, where the average humidity suits them (greater than 50%). However, you can limit your child's exposure to mites by containment measures—confining mites inside their preferred habitats, such as mattresses and pillows with plastic covers—and taking steps to reduce their numbers in places you can't seal off, such as carpets. In chapters 7 and 12 you'll find suggestions for managing dust mites.

Like dust mites, cockroaches are a fact of life almost every place in the world, especially in urban settings. They seem to like living alongside humans, who provide warmth, places to stay, and a nonstop food supply. When they die, their bodies crumble into powder that works its way into the household dust and is breathed into the lungs, promoting allergic inflammation and asthma attacks. A study of inner-city children with asthma found that more than 1 in 3 were sensitive to cockroach proteins. Measures to control roaches are suggested in Chapter 12.

Animals

Contrary to what many people believe, it's not just animal hair or fur that causes asthma and allergies in sensitive youngsters. While hair or fur may be a problem for some, *dander*—the fine scales of dead skin that animals normally shed—and saliva can often be more potent sources of difficulties. Cats and dogs lick people who pat them, thus passing on loads of allergens. They also groom themselves by licking and nibbling, leaving an allergenic saliva coating on their fur.

Finding out that a beloved pet is a trigger for a child's asthma confronts many families with wrenching decisions. The best course—although not a simple or a pleasant one—is to find a new home for the animal. For a child whose asthma is under control with medications and environmental controls, it may be enough to keep the pet permanently outside (see also Chapter 7). Frequent washing and brushing may help to make an animal less allergenic and keep saliva-coated hair and dander from collecting in the household dust, but it is a burden and not always enough to reduce the allergen load.

Small house pets such as mice, rats, rabbits, hamsters, and gerbils are occasional sources of allergens, contributing to the chronic airway inflammation of asthma. If you decide to keep such a pet despite your child's allergies, confine the animal strictly to its cage, clean the cage daily, and keep the cage away from your allergic child's room. A youngster with allergies should not take part in cleaning the cage or caring for the pet. Be sure to let your child's teachers know of your child's animal allergies to avoid difficulties with small animals that are sometimes kept as school residents, or with animals that other children may bring on classroom visits.

Tobacco Smoke

Tobacco smoke is an important and unfortunately prevalent trigger of asthma. Tobacco smoke acts as an irritant that can cause chronic inflammation of the airways, and nudge inflamed airways into constriction and mucus overproduction in a full asthma attack.

Secondhand smoke is dangerous to all children and is a special threat to those with asthma. Don't allow smoking in your home or car and avoid taking your child to homes where people smoke. If your child complains that drivers smoke in school buses during between-trip breaks (the smell is a tip-off), report it to your child's school and to the bus company. If someone in your family still smokes and is finding it hard to quit, urge him to seek medical help—there are a number of useful remedies and approaches to help smokers stop smoking.

Viral Respiratory Infections

Viral infections of the respiratory tract are among the most common childhood illnesses and turn out to be common triggers of airway inflammation and breathing difficulties. In fact, during the cold and flu season, they can be the most important reason children with asthma do poorly, and it is totally unrelated to the problem of allergy. It is believed that viruses responsible for colds, influenza, and other respiratory infections irritate and inflame the airways, making children with asthma do worse. Viral infections may end up stimulating the release of defensive chemicals (see Chapter 1), promoting further inflammation along with the secretion of excessive amounts of protective mucus. A virus that hangs around for several days, as most colds, coughs, and sniffles do, may eventually trigger the typical wheezing and breathing difficulties of an asthma attack.

Lingering aftereffects of viral infections may also interfere with some asthma treatments. Viruses appear to make the bronchi and bronchioles less responsive to inhaled beta-agonist medications for a while, even after the respiratory infection has cleared up.

Emotions

Emotional reactions can sometimes be a trigger for asthma symptoms, but it's a major error to put asthma in the category of emotional or psychological diseases, to suggest it's "all in the mind," or to tell an asthma sufferer to "just get over it." Asthma is an airway disease.

Its symptoms are physical but, like the symptoms of many other conditions, they can be brought on or aggravated by emotional changes. There's also a purely mechanical effect of emotional expression. When a youngster with asthma cries, laughs, or shouts, air flowing faster and harder can further irritate the airway surfaces, triggering bronchoconstriction.

Emotional stress may be relatively important in one youngster's asthma symptoms but less so in another's. If your child needs help getting her asthma and emotions under control, your pediatrician may refer her to an experienced counselor.

Weather

Weather change or extreme weather conditions can affect a child with asthma, but it is not fully understood why. It's speculated that weather changes bring about warm, dry, breezy conditions that blow pollens about and stir up the molds that flourish when it's damp. Rain showers may wash more pollens from trees and grasses, and wind gusts circulate them. Cold air by itself can be a potent asthma trigger. Atmospheric changes during thunderstorms is believed to cause pollen grains to burst and release allergenic particles. When conditions remain unusually still for an extended period, air levels of pollutants can rise to troublesome levels for children with asthma.

Outdoor Air Pollution

Air quality is steadily improving, thanks to government and private initiatives to encourage responsible attitudes toward the environment. However, some degree of air pollution is always going to be the trade-off for the thousands of products and services we depend on.

Chemical gases (eg, ozone, sulfur dioxide, nitrogen oxides) and particles in the air not only irritate the airways and sometimes trigger asthma symptoms, but can also make the airways of a child with asthma more sensitive to his other asthma triggers. People with asthma have increased levels of IgE antibodies (see Chapter 1, page 5) in their lungs after being exposed to diesel fumes and smog, which suggests that pollution may increase a person's reactions to allergens such as pollen and mold. Weather bulletins now routinely include air pollution and ozone advisories. If necessary, keep your child indoors as much as you can when there are smog and ozone alerts (see Chapter 12).

Exercise

Exercise ranks high as an asthma trigger, along with allergies and viral infections. About 80% of people with asthma develop wheezing, coughing, or a tight feeling in the chest when they exercise. The underlying mechanism is not entirely understood. One theory has it that during exercise, a youngster breathes harder and faster, sending a large volume of irritating cold air through the airways and drying out the mucous membranes. Exercise-induced asthma (also known as exercise-induced bronchospasm) usually begins within minutes after a youngster stops exercising and gradually resolves in 30 to 60 minutes, although in some children, asthma symptoms may start a few minutes into exercise.

This doesn't mean that your child with asthma should not take part in sports and strenuous play. On the contrary, youngsters who exercise regularly and control their underlying airway inflammation with medications generally breathe easier and have better health overall. Sports give children with asthma a good way to develop strength and independence. Encourage your child with asthma to take part in any exercise or sport she likes. Some activities may be better tolerated than others. Endurance sports that demand sustained effort without a break may pose a problem for a youngster with asthma. Outdoor sports played on dusty fields may be extra difficult. However, children with asthma can enjoy and excel in swimming, as well as many sports that involve shorter bursts of effort such as baseball, tennis, and cycling. No matter the sport, though, your child should be made aware that athletes with asthma perform at the top level in all sports, including soccer, football, track and field, basketball, and baseball.

Indoor Air Pollution

As homes are made more energy-efficient and better insulated, they can also turn into traps for irritants and allergens that make life uncomfortable for children with asthma. In a "tight" house with double-paned windows and high-grade insulation, air does not flow freely between the indoors and outdoors. Limiting outside air may be an advantage for a child allergic to pollens, but the reduced air circulation can be harmful for a child who is sensitive to fumes from cooking or from a gas or oil furnace, perfumes and air fresheners, aerosol sprays, dust mites, pet dander, and the other allergens found throughout the home. High-efficiency particulate air (HEPA) filters can help clean the air inside the house if they are used in rooms with windows and doors shut. An exhaust hood over the stove can whisk cooking odors and fumes outdoors. Families with asthma may find that life is more comfortable if they eliminate sources of indoor pollution such as wood fires, wood-burning stoves, heavily perfumed soaps and laundry products, and gas ranges (see "An Irritant Hidden in Plain Sight: Nitrogen Dioxide" on page 92). Many aerosol products are available in alternative formulations that are acceptable in allergic households. See Chapter 12 for further suggestions about cutting down on indoor pollution to help your child with asthma.

Medical Triggers for Asthma

Several medical conditions can trigger or worsen asthma symptoms. Treatment of a contributing condition sometimes improves the respiratory problem.

Gastroesophageal Reflux

Occasionally, a child's asthma may be worsened by *reflux,* a backflow problem in the digestive tract. Food normally passes from the mouth through the esophagus, a muscular tube, and into the stomach. A ring of muscle at the base of the esophagus, the lower esophageal sphincter, normally relaxes to let food pass and then tightens again to ensure that the food stays in the stomach, where it is broken down by acids.

An Irritant Hidden in Plain Sight: Nitrogen Dioxide

About half of all homes in the United States have gas-fueled cooking appliances, including ranges and barbecue grills. When gas is burned it gives off *nitrogen dioxide,* a colorless, odorless gas that can interfere with lung function and cause coughing and wheezing. Nitrogen dioxide is released by a pilot light even at times when a gas appliance is not in use. It is also given off by kerosene stoves and heaters.

If you cook with gas, keep your kitchen well ventilated at all times. Budget permitting, install an exhaust fan over the stove with ventilation to the outside. Open the kitchen windows and close the kitchen door to keep fumes out of the rest of the house.

Sometimes, the lower esophageal sphincter opens at the wrong time and lets the acidic stomach contents flow back into the esophagus, where it irritates the delicate membranes lining the esophagus and sometimes goes up high enough to affect the voice box and airways as well. This condition is known as gastroesophageal reflux disease (GERD). It is not the same as the normal, pain-free spitting up of infancy. A child with GERD may complain of a sour taste and a burning sensation in the throat; some, however, have no complaints suggesting reflex. Gastroesophageal reflux disease may aggravate asthma even without the unwanted acid liquid going into the airways, but how this happens is not fully understood. Your pediatrician will examine your child to determine whether GERD is a factor in his asthma. If so, treatment of the digestive problem may also improve the respiratory symptoms.

Sinusitis

Children with chronic or frequent sinusitis (see Chapter 4, page 34) may have asthma that is difficult to control. The exact cause for this is not known. We do know that children with stuffed-up noses caused by sinus congestion tend to breathe through their mouths. Thus, the air they inhale does not undergo the normal warming and moisturization in the nose and sinuses. The large volume of colder air may trigger asthma in inflamed airways just like with exercise-induced asthma (see page 90). Another theory is that when inflamed and infected, the sinuses communicate directly with the bronchi of the lungs, and this results in constriction of the airways. This communication may take place through the pathways of the autonomic nervous system (the nerves that control the heart muscle; the smooth muscles, including those of the airways; and the glands), or it may occur through release by the sinuses of chemical-messenger substances that find their way to the lungs. Treatment of chronic sinusitis may reduce the underlying inflammation and the number of acute asthma attacks (see Chapter 11).

Chapter 10

Asthma in Infants and Toddlers

*D*iagnosing asthma in infants and toddlers is difficult because wheezing and coughing *with respiratory illness at this age can be common. However, information obtained from recent clinical research has been helpful in predicting which wheezy child is likely to go on to have asthma. Once a diagnosis of asthma is made, it can be just as hard to treat the condition given the challenges of effectively delivering medication to a very young child.*

Ever since Danielle was hospitalized at 6 months for a bad case of bronchiolitis, she wheezes every time she catches a cold. Now it is winter and 18-month-old Danielle seems to be catching a cold and wheezing almost every month. The doctor prescribes a nebulizer machine to be used with albuterol and although it makes her jumpy, the treatment improves her symptoms. However, her episodes of wheezing and coughing are happening more often. Twice Danielle needs treatment with oral steroids to get through severe attacks.

The family's pediatrician had initially labeled Danielle's problem "reactive airway disease." However, after confirming a family history of asthma (Danielle's father had asthma problems as a child) and noting how often problems occur, the pediatrician changes the diagnosis to asthma. The parents are not afraid of the new label, as they know that good treatments are available. Danielle's pediatrician prescribes budesonide, an inhaled corticosteroid to be given with the nebulizer with the aim of preventing wheezing attacks.

Thanks to this treatment, the attacks now occur less often and the symptoms are less severe. Danielle's mother gives her the nebulized corticosteroid 2 times a day, even when the toddler is well. She gives albuterol to Danielle by nebulizer only when it's needed. Danielle does not like her "machine" treatments, but her mother has worked out some fun activities to help Danielle cooperate during the treatment.

Which Infants and Toddlers Develop Asthma, and Why?

A rise in asthma cases among infants and toddlers accounts for a large part of the recent overall increase in asthma. For now, we have no satisfactory way to explain the increase in asthma among the very young, although familiar factors common in older age groups—secondhand smoke, dust mites, cockroaches, pet dander—may well play a role. Another explanation may have to do with the "too clean" theory (see "The 'Too Clean' Theory or the 'Hygiene Hypothesis'" in Chapter 4 on page 32).

Wheezing and coughing are common in infants and toddlers, and doctors are cautious about labeling such symptoms as asthma until they have ruled out other possibilities. In the past, however, reluctance to acknowledge that asthma could affect even the youngest children sometimes led to underdiagnosis of asthma. Instead, infants and toddlers were often said to have chronic bronchitis, wheezy bronchitis, reactive airway disease, recurrent pneumonia, or recurrent upper respiratory infections. Consequently, many children with asthma

---

Asthma Predictive Index

Most wheezing during the first 3 years of life is related to viral respiratory infections. Respiratory viruses and symptoms of early asthma may be hard to tell apart, making diagnosis and treatment tricky. But doctors and parents now have a tool to help them predict with reasonable accuracy if the child will develop asthma or simply outgrow it.

The asthma predictive index (API) is a guide to determining which small children will likely have asthma in later years. Children younger than 3 years who have had 4 or more significant wheezing episodes in the past year are much more likely to have persistent (ie, lifelong) asthma after 5 years if they have either of the following:

One major decisive factor
- Parent with asthma
- Physician diagnosis of eczema (atopic dermatitis)
- Sensitivity to allergens in the air (as determined by physician through positive skin tests or blood tests to allergens such as trees, grasses, weeds, molds, or dust mites)

OR

Two minor decisive factors
- Food allergies
- Greater than 4% blood eosinophils (a type of white blood cell often seen in allergic disease)
- Wheezing apart from colds

The API was developed after following almost 1,000 children through 13 years of age. It turned out that a wheezy child with a positive API at around 2 to 3 years of age meant there was about an 80% chance that child would have a definite diagnosis of asthma when entering first grade.

Using the API, doctors and parents can watch more closely for symptoms of asthma as the child grows and if needed, start the right medications earlier. Earlier and better treatment can help keep children active and healthy, and their asthma in good control.

did not get the treatment they needed. Wheezing and coughing are not always symptoms of asthma, but all respiratory symptoms in children should be promptly investigated to determine the cause. From research done on a large number of children followed over many years who go on to develop asthma, there are a few strong indicators that can be used to determine if a wheezy infant or toddler has asthma in the making. It turns out that if there is a history of asthma in the parent of the child, or the child has atopic dermatitis (eczema), the child with recurrent wheezing and breathing difficulties early on in life has a good chance of having a definite diagnosis of asthma in the school-age years (see "Asthma Predictive Index" on the previous page).

Broadly speaking, there are 2 types of wheezing in babies and young toddlers—nonallergic and allergic. Nonallergic infants wheeze only when they have an upper respiratory infection. As these children approach the preschool years, their airways grow larger and the wheezing disappears.

Babies with allergies also wheeze when they catch respiratory viral infections, but unlike the first group, they are likely to develop asthma that will persist throughout childhood and beyond. An important specific type of viral infection early in life often associated with the onset of asthma is respiratory syncytial virus (RSV), which causes bronchiolitis (see "Bronchiolitis" below). Exactly why it appears to trigger a child, particularly an allergy-prone one, to go on to have asthma is not clear. Allergic babies may have other telling signs and symptoms, such as eczema (see Chapter 3), hay fever (allergic rhinitis) (see Chapter 4), or food allergy (see Chapter 5). At this early stage, both groups of wheezers may benefit from asthma treatment. Many in the first group will outgrow the need for medication by about the time they enter kindergarten. Those in the second often continue to require asthma treatment and may need therapy for the other aspects of allergy as well.

Bronchiolitis

Infants and toddlers sometimes have rapid breathing, a deep cough, and loud wheezing 3 to 5 days after developing the typical runny nose and cough of an upper respiratory infection. High fever is often present. This pattern of symptoms can indicate *bronchiolitis,* a viral illness that in some cases is a forerunner of asthma.

If your child's symptoms become more severe or don't start to decrease in the normal 3 to 5 days after she catches a cold or sniffles, consult your pediatrician. In a severe case in which the child looks bluish and has difficulty breathing, call Emergency Medical Services (911 in most areas).

After an initial bout of bronchiolitis, about half of children continue to have recurrent episodes of wheezing when they catch colds or other viral upper respiratory infections. In many cases, wheezing gradually fades away and stops altogether when the child reaches the age of 2 or 3 years. If wheezing persists, it may represent asthma and needs further evaluation by your pediatrician or an asthma specialist.

Babies Have Sensitive Airways

All healthy babies are born with highly responsive airways. This characteristic of infants is similar to the airway hyperresponsiveness that is the hallmark of asthma in older children and adults (see Chapter 1). However, hyperresponsiveness in infants is not a symptom of disease but a normal state that gradually disappears over time unless something interferes with the natural process.

We don't yet know whether or to what extent this early airway responsiveness plays a role in infants' and toddlers' asthma. What we do know is that in normal circumstances, it gradually fades away. In some children, however, exposure to stimuli such as secondhand smoke or certain viral infections, or a family history of asthma, seems to interfere with the process.

It turns out that of all the babies who have recurrent wheezing in their first year, fewer than one-third are still wheezing in later childhood. However, wheezing must always be taken seriously because almost half of all children with asthma develop symptoms before their first birthday.

As a rule, if your infant has 3 or more bouts of significant wheezing, no matter what the cause may be, your pediatrician will consider the possibility of asthma until it can be definitively ruled out. If further evaluation indicates your baby has asthma, your doctor will recommend a treatment plan that includes medications, along with an education program. Your pediatrician will work with you to develop a strategy to prevent severe symptoms and flare-ups.

Diagnosing Asthma in Young Children

One of the difficulties of diagnosing asthma in babies and toddlers is that it's not very easy to measure lung function in small children. So in trying to make a diagnosis, your pediatrician will rely heavily on your child's symptoms and other information. Your pediatrician will ask whether your baby tends to wheeze, cough, or breathe fast when he has a "cold," is near animals, or is in a place that's dusty or tainted by smoke. Make sure you tell your pediatrician about any excessive coughing that your child has, particularly nighttime cough and prolonged cough after a "cold," even if there is no wheezing, because asthma can be present with coughing being the only symptom. Your pediatrician will also ask whether you or other family members have asthma, hay fever, or eczema, or if there's anyone in the family with recurrent bronchitis or sinus problems.

Your pediatrician will listen carefully to make sure that the sounds your baby is making are coming from the airways of the lungs, and not from the baby's voice box higher up in the throat or the nose. Sometimes babies breathe noisily as a result of *laryngotracheomalacia*, a temporary weakness in the cartilage near the vocal cords. They grow out of this as the tissues become firmer. If your baby starts wheezing after breathing in a foreign object (eg, a bit of food, a small toy) that has become lodged in a bronchial tube, he needs urgent medical attention. Unusual conditions related to airway development or prematurity can also cause wheezing in infants. In general, an unexplained frequent cough or daily cough in infants may mean serious disease and should be evaluated by your pediatrician or pediatric pulmonologist.

Your pediatrician will check to make sure your baby is maintaining a satisfactory rate of growth and development. Most infants with asthma make good progress and are otherwise healthy. If your pediatrician is concerned that your baby may be growing too slowly or failing to thrive, tests for conditions other than asthma will be ordered. Certain tests, including a sweat test to rule out cystic fibrosis (see Chapter 2, page 18), may be necessary when your doctor wants to be sure your baby's wheezing and chest symptoms are not caused by a condition with symptoms that are similar to asthma.

Chest radiographs may be ordered during your baby's first wheezing bout to make sure that there isn't a problem in the lungs. If asthma is diagnosed, repeated radiographs are rarely needed because the problem is in the bronchial tubes, which cannot be seen very well in radiographs. Your pediatrician is not likely to recommend allergy testing right away for your baby unless you suspect that wheezing always occurs after your child has been around a certain item, like an animal, or consumed a certain food. However, keep in mind that food allergy is rarely a cause of asthma in infants and toddlers, although it may be a trigger for eczema (see Chapter 3).

Sometimes the easiest and best way to diagnose asthma in a young child is to treat with asthma therapy and see if the child improves. This is because for the most part, medications for asthma only help asthma and not other conditions. If improvement is seen, asthma is the likely diagnosis. If this approach is taken with your child, help your pediatrician by monitoring your child's symptoms carefully so you can give good feedback as to whether the medications have helped.

Reducing Exposure to Asthma Triggers

Babies may develop wheezing when they catch viral respiratory infections—colds and sniffles. In the first year or two, one frequent cause of respiratory illness is a virus known as RSV. Later, rhinoviruses that cause the common cold are the usual suspects. One preventive factor too often overlooked is simple hygiene. Remind family members with colds to dispose of tissues and handkerchiefs properly and to wash their hands frequently with warm water and soap. Ask them to wash their hands before handling your baby. Alcohol-based hand gels are also a good way to help prevent the spread of infections.

Some researchers believe that children who have asthma are more vulnerable to respiratory viruses, but this is not known for sure. All infants and toddlers haven't yet built up immune resistance, so they are particularly susceptible to infections, including respiratory viruses that can injure the airway linings and leave them more vulnerable to inflammation. And when young children with asthma have viral respiratory infections, their asthma often flares up.

The influenza virus is a powerful asthma trigger, and babies older than 6 months who require daily medication for asthma should be given a flu shot every fall. Unlike other immunizations, flu shots are given yearly because the influenza virus continually changes its structure, or mutates, and new vaccines have to be developed to counter the mutations.

Treating Asthma in Infants and Toddlers

In providing a treatment plan for your infant or toddler with asthma, your pediatrician aims for more than simply getting rid of symptoms. A comprehensive treatment plan will encompass the following specific goals:

1. Control symptoms with the fewest medications at the lowest effective doses.
2. Prevent severe asthma episodes.
3. Allow the child to attend child care, play group, and other socializing activities.
4. Permit normal growth and development.
5. Achieve normal activity.
6. Keep side effects of treatment to the lowest possible level.
7. Educate the family and caregivers about asthma and how to manage it.

Treatment for young children, like that for older children and teenagers, comes in 3 parts—education, environmental controls, and medications.

Education

Your pediatrician or asthma specialist will provide information about what asthma is and how it can be effectively controlled. This will include a written action plan that clearly spells out which medications are to be taken for prevention and which are to be used for flare-ups. It should contain information that all caregivers and everyone in the family, including brothers and sisters of all ages, can understand.

Give copies of the asthma information materials and asthma action plan to caregivers, grandparents, and everyone who shares in the care of your child. Take the time to review the materials with them, to make sure they understand what asthma is and how your child's asthma must be managed. Any time your child's treatment plan is revised, send a copy to child care and circulate the new written information among extended family members.

Environmental Controls

In chapters 9 and 12 there are suggestions for reducing your baby's exposure to typical allergens and irritants such as secondhand smoke, fumes and odors, pet dander, dust mites, and cockroaches. Food allergy is unlikely to be the cause of asthma in an infant or toddler;

however, food allergy can sometimes trigger eczema in infancy (see Chapter 3) and is sometimes a forerunner of later asthma and allergies.

Medications

In setting up a treatment plan, your pediatrician aims to gain control over symptoms as quickly as possible, then taper treatment down to the lowest possible dose needed to control symptoms and keep your child active and healthy. Medications are given with the twin goals of long-term control of inflammation and quick relief of symptoms (see Chapter 8, page 79).

Medications given to infants and toddlers are similar to those for older children; only the doses and delivery systems are different. Anti-inflammatory medications are used to control and prevent airway irritability and inflammation. Your doctor may prescribe an inhaled corticosteroid to be given by nebulizer or by an inhaler with spacer (see "Medication Delivery Systems" on page 102). A daily leukotriene modifier medication, given by mouth and swallowed as a granule or chewable tab, is sometimes used in place of an inhaled corticosteroid, or in combination, to help control symptoms. Beta$_2$-agonists (eg, albuterol) are given to relieve symptoms. These medications are given by nebulizer or metered-dose inhaler (MDI) with spacer, or rarely, in the form of syrup.

If your baby has mild asthma symptoms less than twice a week, daily medications probably aren't necessary. Your pediatrician may recommend a medication to open up the airways as needed (eg, albuterol) and will advise you what measures to take if your child catches a respiratory virus or another trigger sets off a bout of symptoms. However, an infant or toddler who has symptoms more than twice a week should be treated on a long-term basis with daily medication to reduce airway inflammation and help ensure long-term asthma control. Sometimes, a daily prevention medication program is recommended for a child who has off-and-on asthma flare-ups that are significant (eg, needs to go to the emergency department, requires oral steroids) and becoming frequent, even though the child may be entirely asthma-free for a period between flare-ups.

At all times, your pediatrician will monitor your child's progress closely and adjust treatment as appropriate. When your child has done well over an extended period, your pediatrician may recommend a step-down, reducing the dosage to see if control can be maintained with less medication or a different dosing schedule. If your child has mainly seasonal asthma (eg, fall, winter), sometimes taking him off his controller medication for a period, like during the summer, can be tried. Discuss this possibility with your pediatrician; don't do it on your own. If this is not possible with your child, there is good news—studies have shown that asthma medications at correct doses are safe for long-term use.

> ## Croup
>
> A young child who wakes in the middle of the night with a barking, seal-like cough and trouble breathing may have *croup.* Occasionally, croup and asthma can be confused. Usually caused by a mild upper respiratory infection or sometimes by allergy, croup is an inflammation of the voice box (larynx) and windpipe (trachea). It causes swelling that narrows the airway just below the vocal cords and makes breathing noisy and difficult. Asthma, by contrast, is a problem with the airways much farther down—in the bronchi.
>
> Boys get croup more often than girls. Children rarely get croup after about age 4 years.
>
> A croup attack usually eases if the child breathes for 15 to 20 minutes in a warm, steamy bathroom or next to a open window letting in cool air. Your pediatrician may suggest that you use a cool-mist humidifier in your child's room for a few nights.
>
> If the child is sick enough to have to go to the office or hospital emergency department, sometimes an injectable steroid is given or a few days of an oral steroid is prescribed, to reduce the inflammation. Medical attention is needed if croup symptoms are unusually severe. Go to the nearest hospital emergency department promptly if
>
> - Your child can't speak for lack of breath.
> - Your child is struggling to breathe despite treatment at home.

Medication Delivery Systems

It's difficult to give medications to infants and toddlers—they're small, their coordination is still developing, and they can't be expected to follow complicated directions. The best way to get medication into airways is to inhale it in directly, but this is not easy to do with young children. One method used is with a *nebulizer machine,* an electrical appliance that converts liquid medication in to a fine mist. Your pediatrician or asthma specialist may suggest an MDI (commonly referred to as an inhaler) that is used in conjunction with a spacer device.

It's very important to use a nebulizer correctly to make sure your child gets an adequate and correct dose of medication. A mask is used for infants and young toddlers. The mask must be held close to the face, covering the mouth and nose; holding it away from the face and using a blow-by technique is not advised—too much medication is lost into the air. When a child is old enough, convert from mask to using a mouthpiece, whereby the medication is inhaled directly in via the mouth; doing this results in more of the dose reaching the lungs.

If your child is taking inhaled medication using an MDI with a spacer device, including a mask, it is essential the mask is fitted tightly to the face, surrounding the nose and mouth. Without this, leakage around the mask occurs, resulting in much less delivered medication to the lungs. When 2 doses or puffs are used, make sure each puff is fired and inhaled, one at a time.

If your child attends in-home child care, a child care center, a play group, or a nursery school, make sure there is a medically trained caregiver who knows how to use your child's medication delivery device. Demonstrate to this person(s) how your child takes the inhaled medication, when it is to be used, and any tricks you've learned to help get it done successfully. Try to leave an extra set of inhaled medication and delivery devices with the caregiver so as to avoid having to drop off the items each day.

Chapter 11

Asthma Treatments

*N*ew treatments and a deeper understanding of the mechanisms behind asthma *enable pediatricians to greatly help youngsters and adults control the condition. With the right medications and instructions for their use, children with asthma can prevent daily symptoms and prevent progression of exacerbations that lead to emergency care visits and hospitalization. Those with asthma should be able to stay active, prevent severe symptoms, and avoid emergency trips to the hospital. Although asthma is a major cause of emergency care and hospitalization, these unhappy events can be prevented by good medical care.*

Tyler has always had a tendency to have "chest colds," but when the 7-year-old ends up in the emergency department with wheezing and difficulty breathing, the emergency physician says that asthma is more likely his problem.

A week after the emergency visit, Tyler's pediatrician checks the youngster's pulmonary function. It is lower than normal. He also has Tyler fill out an asthma control test, and he fails it, indicating poor control. When the pediatrician learns that Tyler is missing a fair number of school days because of breathing problems and is less active than other children, he prescribes an inhaled corticosteroid controller medication, selecting an age-appropriate delivery device from among the various available. The pediatrician tells Tyler's mother that the boy should take the medication every day, shows Tyler how to use the device, and has Tyler demonstrate successful use. The doctor reassures Tyler and his mom that inhaled steroids are very effective and safe medications for preventing the daily symptoms of chronic asthma.

Is the Treatment Working?

You can be confident that asthma treatment is working when your child or teenager
- Doesn't miss school days.
- Regularly sleeps through the night.
- Participates normally and fully in sports and play.
- Is not having to use albuterol (ie, quick-relief medication) often.

If any of these 4 elements is lacking or not fully addressed, the youngster's asthma is not properly under control and the treatment needs to be revised.

The doctor also refers Tyler to a pediatric allergy specialist, who takes a careful environmental history and conducts skin tests and finds that Tyler has allergy antibodies to indoor (eg, dust mite, cat, indoor molds) and outdoor (eg, pollens, outdoor molds) allergens. He also carries out a pulmonary function test on Tyler, which shows his lung function is pretty close to normal now that he is on his daily controller medication.

The allergy specialist suggests ways Tyler's family can modify his environment to reduce allergy triggers. Measures include dust mite control in his bedroom and finding a good loving home for the cat. The doctor works out an asthma action plan that provides instructions for what preventive measures need to be done daily and what extra measures are to be started when symptoms do not respond fully to occasional use of his bronchodilator (albuterol). This includes starting oral steroids for a few days if his asthma is doing poorly and aggressive bronchodilator therapy is not working. At subsequent 3-month regular checkups, Tyler and his mother have lots to be proud of. By following through with the asthma program, Tyler has not missed a single day in the school year, is overall more active, and is enjoying normal play and sports.

$\mathcal{T}$he treatment of children's asthma is a three-way partnership. It requires equal participation from the doctor, the child with asthma, and the child's family. While your child is an infant or toddler, you as the parent will be in charge of his treatment. As he grows into the preschool years, however, encourage him to take increasing responsibility. This will start to prepare him for the time when, as a young adult, he will be a partner in a two-way treatment alliance with his doctor. In setting up a treatment plan for your child, your physician aims for the following specific goals:

1. Treatment should calm the inflamed airways to prevent troublesome chronic symptoms, such as coughing and breathlessness at night or after exercise.
2. By keeping airway inflammation and twitchiness under control, treatment should enable the child to breathe freely and maintain normal lung function.
3. The child should be able to keep up with his friends and schoolmates in sports, play, and other activities.
4. Treatment should prevent periodic worsening of asthma and virtually eliminate the need for emergency department visits or admissions to the hospital.
5. Prescribed medications should be easy to use and provide good symptom control with a low rate of side effects.

When the child and family fulfill their roles in the treatment partnership, it should control asthma as well as or even better than they expected at the start of therapy.

Asthma Can Change; So Must Treatment

Because asthma can change from time to time, the way your child's asthma is managed may need to be adjusted periodically. Medication doses may need to go up or, conversely, decreased (which can be viewed as good news). This is why it is important to keep in frequent touch with your pediatrician and report any change that may suggest the need for fine-tuning. Follow-up visits will be recommended by your child's physician—don't skip them just because your child's asthma is doing well.

Proper treatment usually involves

- Environmental or behavioral measures to minimize exposure to asthma triggers
- Medications to control chronic airway inflammation, if felt to be present, and to relieve acute symptoms early on before they progress to the point of requiring an unscheduled medical visit
- Depending on the age of the child and severity of the asthma, the use of a peak flow meter to see how well your child's lungs are functioning
- Regular follow-up in the office or clinic, monitoring how well the child's asthma is under control, and checking pulmonary function (if the child is old enough to do this) at intervals to ensure that persistent airway obstruction is not present

A Written Treatment Plan

Your child's pediatrician or asthma specialist will ask you and your child how often symptoms come on and how severe they are. Then, after performing lung-function tests and determining how severe your child's asthma is, your doctor will probably prepare a specific written asthma treatment plan for your child (see Chapter 10, page 100). A treatment plan is a stepwise medication approach keyed to your child's symptoms, peak flow meter readings, or both, which will enable you to adjust the medications to stop symptoms from worsening.

Your physician may start medications at a higher level to get airway inflammation under control, then carefully reduce the dosage or the number of medications until treatment arrives at the lowest dose needed to maintain control. With this approach, asthma can best be brought under control and medication side effects kept to a manageable level.

Peak Flow Meter

A *peak flow meter* (or, rarely, a small electronic portable spirometer) is sometimes recommended as part of a treatment plan. These handheld devices measure how fast a person can blow air out of the lungs. Asthma causes patients to not be able to blow air out fast because their airways are narrowed, so a low measurement with this device suggests problems are occurring with your child's asthma. These measurements can help warn a patient or parent that extra medication is needed to fend off more severe asthma symptoms. The results can also be useful for the patient who does not adequately perceive worsening airway obstruction or who has difficulty distinguishing anxiety or hyperventilation attacks from asthma. When your child is having asthma problems, a peak flow reading puts a number on how she is doing, much as a thermometer shows how high a temperature is. Your pediatrician or asthma specialist will show you how to record your child's baseline measurements (see "How to Use a Peak Flow Meter" on the next page) at a time when she is doing well with her asthma. This is referred to as her "personal best." When your child's asthma is not doing well or is at risk of flaring up (eg, during a "cold"), a peak flow reading can be obtained and the value compared to the child's personal best. Using a simple range of color zones—green, yellow, and red, like traffic lights—specific recommendations can be spelled out as to what needs to be done to prevent a full-blown asthma attack based on what color zone the patient falls into with her peak flow measurement.

How to Use a Peak Flow Meter

Your child's peak flow–based asthma treatment plan uses his own personal best peak flow reading because every child is unique. Your child's peak flow may be higher or lower than that of another child even though their age, sex, and height are identical.

To find your child's personal best, your pediatrician will instruct him to use the peak flow meter at the same time every day for 2 to 3 weeks during a period when he doesn't have any symptoms and asthma is under good control.

To obtain a peak flow measurement, have your child do the following:

1. Stand up.

2. Place the peak flow device indicator at 0.

3. Take a deep breath, then place the device well in to the mouth.

4. Close his lips around the mouthpiece and keep his tongue clear of the opening.

5. Blow once as hard and fast as he can. Note the reading.

Repeat steps 2 through 5 twice more and write down the highest score.

After your child has established his personal best your doctor may ask him to use the meter for readings when he is beginning to have symptoms, or when he has a "cold" (a time when asthma commonly gets worse). The doctor may also ask you to monitor his peak flow when adjustments have been made to his medication program, whether it be up or down, to detect any change in asthma control.

Starting at about age 4 or 5 years, your child can learn how to use a peak flow meter. The following color zone system is commonly used with peak flow monitoring:

- Green means that the airflow score is at 80% to 100% of your child's personal best peak flow (the targeted peak flow value determined by your child's pediatrician); his medications don't need to be adjusted and he may continue full activity.
- Yellow means *caution,* just as it does on the road with a traffic light; airflow is between 50% and 80% of your child's personal best and certain additional asthma medications should be started or increased to ward off symptoms.
- Red means *danger;* your child's score is less than 50% of his peak flow. Have your child take his quick-relief medications (usually a bronchodilator at a high dose to open up the airways and steroid pills or liquid to calm inflammation) if it is part of the asthma action plan worked out between you and your pediatrician or asthma specialist. Call or see your physician soon, or go for emergency care, if the peak flow reading stays below 50% despite the treatment.

The peak flow meter provides one way to measure asthma objectively, but it's critical that the child and everyone else in the family not rely on just a peak flow number for assessment of how a child's asthma is doing. Symptoms are as important, probably even more important, than a peak flow reading. It is not uncommon for symptoms to detect a flare-up of asthma even before peak flow measurements do.

Environmental Controls

It is important to identify your child's allergic asthma triggers, if possible. This is sometimes done with the help of allergy skin tests or blood tests (see Chapter 9). Once the results are known, the next important step is to remove or reduce as many allergens from your home as you can (see chapters 9 and 12). It's impossible to make the place you live in completely allergen-free, but you can at least reduce their number. Studies have shown that reducing the levels of allergens can make a significant improvement in asthma symptoms after a period as short as 2 weeks.

Medications

Asthma medications are given for long-term control and quick relief. Long-term control medications are used to calm airway inflammation and control the symptoms of chronic asthma. They include anti-inflammatory agents (eg, corticosteroids), sometimes with the addition of long-acting bronchodilators, and leukotriene modifiers. Quick-relief medications (previously called "rescue medication"; this term is no longer used because it is not an accurate description) are short-acting beta$_2$-agonists (eg, albuterol) given to stop acute tightening of the airways and airway blockage (see Table 11-1 on page 114). Sometimes this distinction between controller and quick-relief medication can be blurry because albuterol is commonly used before exercise and running to prevent exercise-induced asthma, and oral corticosteroids are given for a few days to quickly relieve an acute asthma attack.

Corticosteroids and Growth

Concerns have been raised that inhaled corticosteroids may slow children's growth when used over a long period, but physicians believe that when treatment is properly conducted, corticosteroids do not have an adverse effect on the final height children attain. By contrast, chronic asthma that is poorly controlled is known to slow the growth rate and delay physical maturation in some children. Your doctor will prescribe corticosteroids at the lowest effective dose and monitor your child's growth rate at regular checkups. Regular monitoring of growth by your physician is of value in identifying any slowing of growth.

Long-term Control

Corticosteroids
Synthetic versions of hormones produced in the adrenal glands, corticosteroids are the most powerful anti-inflammatory medications now available for treating asthma. In inhaled form, they are used exclusively for long-term control; they are not very effective for acute symptoms. Systemic corticosteroids taken by mouth as pills or liquid, or injected, are sometimes of value to get asthma quickly under control when a child is beginning long-term asthma therapy. Inhaled corticosteroids are the agents preferred and recommended as first-line treatment of chronic asthma by various asthma expert panels that publish guidelines on the proper treatment of asthma. They are available in various forms and different dosage forms, which make them convenient for patients to take, such as an aerosol in a metered-dose inhaler (MDI), a dry powder inhaler (DPI), and a liquid form that can be used in a nebulizer for small children.

Leukotriene Modifiers
These compounds act by decreasing the effects of an inflammatory chemical made by the body known as *leukotrienes*. The 2 leukotriene modifiers currently in use, montelukast and zafirlukast, are used as control medications. They have only mild to moderate beneficial effects at best but are very safe. They are taken in pill form; chewable and sprinkle forms are available for young children.

Long-Acting Beta$_2$-Agonists
Medications in the beta$_2$-agonist class work by relaxing the muscles that wrap around the bronchi of the lungs and tend to squeeze down and narrow the airways in those who have asthma. The short-acting forms of beta$_2$-agonists, such as albuterol, are used as first-line agents for relief of asthma in all patients with asthma. Long-acting versions of beta$_2$-agonists were made by making some chemical changes in the short-acting beta$_2$-agonists. These long-acting beta$_2$-agonists are almost always prescribed together with anti-inflammatory medications for long-term control, rarely if ever by themselves. They are usually added when a conventional dose of an inhaled steroid is not adequate for control of daily symptoms.

There is evidence that rare patients experience loss of effect from their rapid-acting bronchodilator (eg, albuterol, levalbuterol) with taking long-acting bronchodilators. While this is quite uncommon, patients should be advised of this potential and instructed to notify their physician if the addition of a long-acting bronchodilator is associated with increased symptoms instead of the usual increased benefit.

Theophylline

Theophylline, usually taken by mouth as a timed-release pill, opens up the airways for an extended period. It can be used alone or together with inhaled corticosteroids. It can be particularly helpful in preventing nighttime symptoms in mild to moderate asthma. Although once used extensively, theophylline is currently infrequently prescribed for asthma, mainly because it requires careful monitoring of blood levels to avoid side effects and because other asthma medications often work as well or better.

Cromolyn Sodium and Nedocromil

These are very mildly effective anti-inflammatory medications rarely used anymore in long-term therapy of mild to moderate asthma in children.

Quick Relief

Short-Acting Beta$_2$-Agonists

These are used for the rapid relief of acute asthma symptoms and to prevent exercise-induced asthma in children. They are first-line treatment of acute asthma symptoms—all patients with asthma need to have available a short-acting beta$_2$-agonist. Children may use them by MDI or nebulizer; either form is effective if used properly. The medication should be available at home, in school, and at the site of sports participation. This class of medication used to be called "rescue" medicine, but this term is no longer used because it implies that a patient must be in terrible shape to use it, which should not be the case. The new preferred term is *quick relief.* It turns out that almost all patients use albuterol (or a close cousin called levalbuterol, which acts very similar to albuterol) for their quick-relief medication. Albuterol should be used for any asthma symptom, including wheeze, chest tightness, and cough, and not just reserved for asthma attacks.

Anticholinergics

Ipratropium bromide, a rapid-acting bronchodilator, may be used as an alternative to dilate the airways when inhaled beta$_2$-agonists cannot be used, or given together with an inhaled beta$_2$-agonist in severe asthma.

Systemic Corticosteroids

These are given by mouth or injection to reduce inflammation inside the airways and speed recovery when a youngster is having an asthma flare-up.

Medication Delivery Systems

Asthma medications can be inhaled directly into the lungs or taken systemically (ie, by ingestion or injection). Inhalation using an MDI or nebulizer has a number of advantages over other routes of taking medication, the major one being that the medication passes straight into the airways, reducing or avoiding side effects altogether as a result. In addition, with at least bronchodilator medications, taking the medicine by inhalation has a much faster effect than when taken by mouth. The advantage of taking corticosteroids by inhalation is that they work topically within the airways and as a result have fewer, if any, side effects than when given by mouth.

Several different types of handheld inhalers are on the market; your pediatrician or asthma specialist will suggest the one most suitable for your child. There are important differences in the way they are used and in the amounts of medication they deliver to airways. Your child should be taught how to use the inhaler most suitable for him, and his inhaler technique should be checked regularly to make sure the correct dose of medication is being delivered (see "How to Use a Metered-Dose Inhaler" and "How to Use a Dry Powder Inhaler" on page 117). You pediatrician may prescribe a nebulizer machine in addition to or in place of an MDI, to be used at home for inhaling asthma medication. You will be asked to put a liquid medication into the nebulizer bowl and have your child inhale a fine mist over a period of minutes. As with an MDI, it is essential you know how to use the nebulizer correctly so your child gets the most out of the treatment (see Table 11-2 on page 116).

Table 11-1. Asthma Medications

Medication	Why Used	Possible Side Effects	Comments
Corticosteroids (Glucocorticoids)		Cough, hoarseness, oral thrush (yeast infection)	Safe when properly used
Inhaled • Beclomethasone dipropionate • Budesonide • Mometasone • Fluticasone propionate • Ciclesonide	• Long-term symptom prevention; control of inflammation • Reduce need for oral steroids • Reduce need for albuterol	When given in high doses for too long, may affect growth and have effects on bones and skin.	Different corticosteroids are not interchangeable and must be used under pediatrician's close supervision.
Systemic • Methylprednisolone • Prednisolone • Prednisone • Dexamethasone	For short-term burst to get persistent asthma under control	Appetite change, weight gain, mood change; if given in high doses for too long, may affect growth, and may cause many other serious side effects.	Need to start sufficiently early in the course of an asthma flare-up to prevent hospitalizations and emergency visits.
Long-Acting Beta$_2$-Agonists *Inhaled* • Salmeterol • Formoterol	Long-term symptom prevention, when added to inhaled corticosteroid	• Palpitations, tremor, jittery feeling. • Treatment effect may slightly weaken in long-term treatment, but still effective medications.	• Not to be used in place of anti-inflammatory medication. • Should be used in conjunction with inhaled corticosteroids. • May ensure better symptom control when added to inhaled corticosteroid (instead of increasing steroid dose).
Long-Acting Beta$_2$-Agonist/ Inhaled Corticosteroid Combination • Salmeterol/ fluticasone • Formoterol/ budesonide • Formoterol/ mometasone	• Long-term control and prevention • Reduce/ prevent inflammation and prevent bronchospasm	Same as for long-acting beta$_2$-agonists and inhaled corticosteroids (see above)	Often prescribed when a single agent (eg, inhaled corticosteroid) is not adequate for control
Leukotriene Modifiers • Montelukast • Zafirlukast • Zileuton	Long-term control and prevention given as a single medication or in combination with others	Low rate of side effects	Once-a-day dosing by mouth is convenient (montelukast).

Table 11-1. Asthma Medications *(continued)*

Medication	Why Used	Possible Side Effects	Comments
Mast Cell Stabilizers • Cromolyn sodium • Nedocromil	Long-term symptom prevention or preventive treatment before exercise or known allergen exposure	These medications have virtually no side effects. Some patients dislike taste of nedocromil.	• Rarely prescribed. • Of historical interest only. • Safety is the major advantage of these medications.
Theophylline	Long-term control and prevention of symptoms	Stimulation, jitteriness, sleeplessness, stomach troubles, increased hyperactivity in some children	• Treatment may require careful monitoring of blood levels to guard against side effects. • Not generally used for worsening of symptoms. • Usually an add-on or second-tier medication.
Short-Acting Inhaled Beta$_2$-Agonists • Albuterol • Levalbuterol • Pirbuterol • Terbutaline (These are available as metered-dose inhaler, solution for nebulizer, or liquid and tablets to take by mouth.)	• Quick relief for acute symptoms • Preventive use before exercise	Racing heart, tremor, jittery feeling	• In general, inhaled medications act faster and with fewer side effects than those given by other routes. • Not for regular daily use. • If use increases (eg, if need to use for symptoms more often than 2–3 days per week), asthma may not be properly controlled; control medication should be started or increased. • Levalbuterol is an alternative form of albuterol, which may be associated with decreased side effects. Either agent is equally effective at treating acute asthma symptoms.
Anticholinergic Ipratropium bromide	• Relieves acute bronchospasm. • May decrease mucus secretion.	Dry mouth, drying of respiratory secretions	Used mainly in emergency department for acute asthma not responsive to albuterol alone

New treatments for asthma are always under development. This table includes the range available in September 2010; however, your pediatrician will tell you about new medications and delivery systems as they become available.

Table 11-2. Medication Delivery Devices

Device and Medication	Who Can/Should Use It	How to Use It	Comments
Metered-Dose Inhaler (MDI) • Beta$_2$-agonists • Corticosteroids • Corticosteroid/ long-acting beta-agonist • Cromolyn sodium • Nedocromil • Anticholinergics	All infants and children	• Actuate while taking a slow, deep breath for 3–5 seconds; hold breath for 10 seconds. • Should be used with spacer in young children; not always necessary with older children.	• Difficult to coordinate firing of device with inhalation; spacer helps with this. • Rinse mouth after corticosteroid to reduce amount absorbed by swallowing and topical effect in the mouth and throat.
Breath-Actuated MDI Beta$_2$-agonists	Children older than 6 years	Use device while inhaling for 3–5 seconds, then hold breath for 10 seconds.	• Suitable for children who have difficulty coordinating MDI use with breathing. • Only available as Maxair Autohaler.
Dry Powder Inhaler (DPI) • Long-acting beta$_2$-agonists • Corticosteroids	• Results are more consistent in children older than 6 years. • May be used by some children as young as age 4 or 5 years.	Rapid, deep, forceful breath in 1–2 seconds	• The child must breathe in hard and fast. • Rinse mouth to reduce amount absorbed by swallowing.
Spacer/Holding Chamber Used together with an MDI	• Any child who needs help using an MDI. • Children younger than 4 years should use with valved holding chamber with tight-fitting face mask.	• Actuate MDI into spacer; immediately inhale slowly (3–5 seconds) and deeply; or with face mask, infant or young child to breathe normally for 5–6 breaths. • Actuate only once into spacer/chamber per inhalation.	• Easier to use than MDI alone. • With face mask, enables small children to use MDI. • Can increase dose of medication delivered to lungs. • Decreases amount of dose left in back of throat and reduces absorption through swallowing.
Nebulizer • Beta$_2$-agonists • Anticholinergics • Corticosteroids	• Young children who cannot use MDI with valved holding chamber and face mask • Any child not getting enough benefit from MDI	• Slow, regular breathing with occasional deep breaths • Tightly fitting face mask for children who cannot use mouthpiece	• Easy to use • Relatively expensive; time-consuming and no more effective for most than an MDI with or without spacer

How to Use a Metered-Dose Inhaler

Your child must use her metered-dose inhaler (MDI) correctly to get the right dose of medication. Check that she follows steps 1 through 7 every time she uses her inhaler.

1. Remove cap, hold inhaler upright, and shake it.

2. Tilt head back a little and slowly breathe out.

3. Place inhaler as shown in A (open mouth technique), B (closed mouth technique), or C (with a spacer). Your doctor will tell you which of these 3 techniques to use for your child.

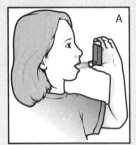 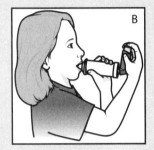 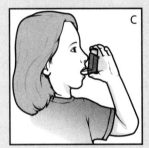

4. Without spacer: Press down on inhaler to release medication right after starting to breathe in. With spacer: Press down on inhaler to release medication into the spacer, and soon after, start to breathe in.

5. Breathe in slowly for 3 to 5 seconds.

6. Hold breath for 10 seconds to let medication reach into lungs.

7. Repeat puff according to your doctor's instructions.

Using a valved holding chamber with a mask (not shown here) can be useful for young children. A different technique is required for this; talk with your pediatrician about it.

How to Use a Dry Powder Inhaler

A dry powder inhaler (DPI) is used a little differently from a metered-dose inhaler (MDI).

1. Load the device. There are a number of DPI-type devices; each has a different way of loading the medication before inhaling it. Know the directions for the device your child is using.

2. Tilt head back a little and slowly breathe out, away from the device.

3. Place the DPI well into mouth as shown in D. Make sure the device is held horizontal and it is headed straight back toward the throat, not angled up or down.

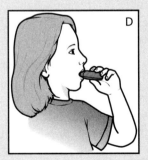

4. The child's lips should be tightly sealed around the mouthpiece of the device.

5. Breathe in rapidly and forcefully (different from how to inhale with an MDI, which is slowly).

6. Hold breath for 10 seconds (although a long breath hold with a DPI is not as important as with an MDI).

7. Repeat puff according to your doctor's instructions.

Tips to Prevent Inhaler Mistakes

- Breathe in through the mouth, not the nose.

- Press down on a metered-dose inhaler (MDI) (without spacer) right after the start of breathing in, but not too late into the inhalation. When used with a spacer, wait for the MDI to be fired first, then immediately start breathing in.

- Breathe in slowly when using an MDI. In contrast, breathe in rapidly when using a dry powder inhaler (DPI).

- Use one puff at a time with an MDI (one puff/one breath). Do not fire the MDI more than once for each breathing in.

- Do not breath out into a DPI device—it can cause a loss of that dose.

- Try to breathe in evenly and deeply.

- Hold breath for at least 10 seconds. Don't cheat!

- Clean and maintain the device exactly as the manufacturer's written instructions tell you.

- Many MDIs and DPIs have dose counters; if so, always check the counter to see how much medication is left in the device.

Asthma at School

In schools, quick-relief medication (eg, albuterol, levalbuterol) should be available in the school office for as-needed purposes. For children who are mature enough to keep their own medications and use them responsibly (usually around age 8 years), they should be permitted to self-carry their albuterol or levalbuterol. All 50 states and the District of Columbia now have laws protecting a student's right to carry and administer asthma medications. A note from the doctor's office stating a child can self-carry (in pocket, fanny pack, or backpack) will likely be necessary, or a school form will need to be filled out. Having a backup inhaler in the nurses office is a good idea for the child who self-carries, just in case the child forgets to bring his inhaler to school. Don't forget—children need to also have their quick-relief medication available when they go on field trips.

Physicians treating school-aged children with asthma need to prepare a written plan to be sent to each child's school. If your child's pediatrician does not, ask for a written plan that covers

- A strategy to manage worsening symptoms, including an action plan to make sure the child can quickly get to his medications and, when appropriate, a recommendation that he be allowed to take his own medications as needed
- An explanation of the medications the child uses for long-term control
- Measures to prevent exercise-induced asthma
- Identification of all of the student's known allergens and asthma triggers

Your child's pediatrician or asthma specialist will probably recommend that daily, long-term medications, when needed, be taken at home, not at school. Therefore, only quick-relief medication is usually needed at school. Any time your child's asthma action plan is revised, send a copy, along with a supply of the new medications and directions, to the school nurse.

Adolescence

As children enter adolescence, asthma may be one of the many factors that cause conflicting feelings about their emerging independence. At this stage, many find it difficult to accept that asthma is a lifelong condition that requires lifelong—perhaps daily—treatment. They may see an asthma treatment plan as an intrusion on their freedom to choose and act for themselves as they see fit. Adolescence is a time of life when the child feels invincible; because of this, the adolescent may want to stop taking any preventive medication for asthma. The parent has to make a special effort to monitor whether this is happening; if it is, solving the problem needs to occur in a skillful fashion whereby the child does not rebel further, worsening the situation.

Your teenager's move toward independence should include more direct interaction with the pediatrician or asthma specialist about health care decisions. This kind of involvement helps your teenager build a positive self-image and assume increasing responsibility; your teen's pediatrician may even suggest seeing the teen without parents present. Doing this allows for setting treatment goals important to the child, and working out an acceptable treatment plan the child is willing to realistically follow. The doctor may invite you to join in and review the plan at the end of the visit, emphasizing your role in supporting your child's efforts.

Athletes and Asthma

Children with asthma benefit from taking part in sports and physical activity and should be encouraged to do so. One of the goals of asthma treatment is to enable youngsters to take part in activities they enjoy without being hampered by asthma symptoms. Of course, your child may benefit from your guidance in making a reasonable choice of activity that doesn't result in disappointment or failure because of a high level of associated allergens and asthma triggers. In most cases, exercise-induced asthma can be prevented by taking medication, such as albuterol, just before the exercise activity. Children who have only minor symptoms with exercise can sometimes prevent them altogether with a lengthy warm-up, instead of taking medication.

Exercise to keep a person from becoming overweight is particularly important when it comes to asthma. Overweight children have a higher incidence of asthma than others, tend to have more severe disease, and have more frequent emergency visits to doctors and hospitals. Children who are told not to exercise because of asthma become *deconditioned* (out of shape) and may ultimately have difficulty distinguishing between real breathing problems from asthma and those that come from the normal shortness of breath of exercise. This is why it is so important that asthma not get in the way of a child being able to run, play, and burn calories while doing it.

Let teachers and coaches know in writing that your child has exercise-induced asthma and may need to use an inhaler before sports. Children who perform competitively at a high level need to talk to their physicians and coaches about medications and prevention strategies in line with the standards set by the US Olympic Committee.

If symptoms come on while a child is playing at her usual activity level, her long-term preventive treatment may need to be revised. Only in rare cases, where a child has severe asthma or another condition, is it necessary to limit participation in sports. Children who exercise regularly are more fit and better able to deal with asthma than those who are inactive and out of shape. Exercise-induced shortness of breath despite using a pre-exercise bronchodilator, and excellent control of a child's asthma otherwise, suggest some other cause and warrant further evaluation by your pediatrician or asthma specialist.

Complementary Therapies

People with asthma sometimes use "natural" therapies to treat their condition. Words that describe these therapies include *alternative, complementary,* and *folk remedy.* Many find these treatments comforting, and in most cases, they may do no harm as long as they are not used in place of the medications and other measures recommended by your child's pediatrician. If you've made the decision to seek natural therapies for your child's care, involve your pediatrician in the process. Your doctor may be able to help you better understand these therapies, whether they have scientific merit, whether claims about them are accurate or exaggerated, and whether they pose any risks to your child's well-being. Keep in mind that a "natural" treatment does not always mean a "safe" one. Your pediatrician can help you determine whether there is a risk of interactions with your child's other medications.

PART 4

LIFESTYLE, THE ENVIRONMENT, AND ASTHMA

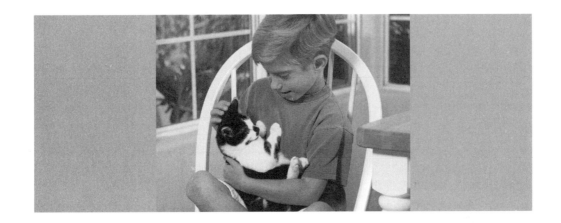

Chapter 12

Environmental and Lifestyle Factors

*I*s there a furry pet in your home? Does a member of the household smoke? Is your child overweight? And what about all that carpeting?

A big part of asthma control involves identifying environmental and lifestyle asthma triggers and acting to minimize their effects. This means looking for potential culprits in your home. It also means examining your lifestyle for factors that may be adding to the problem.

Asthma is a chronic lung disease that can range in severity from mild to severe. The frequency of asthma attacks can vary over time, even in the same individual. For those patients with symptoms occurring many times a week, or asthma attacks that awaken them from sleep or affect regular activities, daily medication is required. Some families may dislike having to take a daily medication or may not recognize the importance of preventive asthma care. Instead, they resort to a crisis management approach, which asthma experts say is the worst way to treat the condition.

The Gibbons family is a good example. Mom and Dad work full-time to make ends meet. Two of their 3 children have asthma; Adam, their 5-year-old, has it the worst. The family carries health insurance, but it's not great—they have a high-deductible plan for the family to be able to afford the cost of the insurance coverage.

Adam has had so many urgent care visits to the local hospital emergency department (ED) that the staff know him by name. The bills from the ED are piling up. Mom is about to lose her job because of all the time off she has had to take to deal with the care of her son's asthma. It has been hard for the family to do the follow-up visit with their pediatrician recommended by the ED because it means more time off of work, and Adam has to be taken out of school. The cost of asthma medications is high, and sometimes Mom decides she is going to see if Adam can go without his recommended preventive medications to help save money, hoping he won't need them anymore. But then he ends up back in the ED.

Finally, Mom hears about a pediatric clinic that takes care of a lot of children with asthma, so the family starts to use this clinic for care. They are open on Saturdays, which helps a lot, and unlike previous care, Mom and Adam see the same doctor for his checkups. Adam and his parents learn about the importance of preventive medication and the need to take it daily because it helps reduce the need for other medications when his asthma goes out of control. This is something they previously did not understand. They receive a specific asthma action plan that spells out the steps and measures to follow to keep Adam's asthma in check. This includes information about what to do when his asthma worsens, with the important goal of keeping Adam out of the ED. Adam and his family are referred to a special asthma disease management program conducted by the local American Lung Association chapter, where they learn about the importance of keeping their home free of asthma triggers. They work diligently in the house on keeping the levels of dust mite, mold, and cockroach to a minimum in order to help out Adam. Dad, who is a smoker, agrees to stop, wanting to do everything he can for his son, and joins a smoke-cessation support group. The parents learn about a pharmaceutical company patient-assistance program that helps reduce the cost of Adam's asthma medications and helps with their ability and willingness to give Adam his daily medications.

Four months later, Adam has had no ED visits, is regularly attending school, and is playing in a soccer league—something he wasn't able to do before because his asthma wouldn't allow all the exercise and running. Although still struggling with all the bills, the Gibbons don't have the large medical expenses they were having before.

. . . .

*A*sthma is one of the most common chronic diseases among American children, affecting more than 6 million. There are many families like the Gibbons in which asthma takes a huge toll. It is one of the most frequent causes for children being admitted to hospitals and accounts for more than 2 million visits to pediatricians each year. It is estimated that children miss more than 12 million school days because of asthma. When all the costs are added up, it's no wonder that this single disease costs the United States $19.7 billion a year in hospitalizations, doctor visits, medications, and loss of workdays.

Asthma: Nature + Nurture

The numbers of children in the United States estimated to have asthma vary from 4 to almost 10 out of every 100, depending on who's counting. Even at the lower estimate, the numbers are too high. But why these kids? What is known about their genetics, environment, and lifestyle that puts them at risk to develop asthma, and once they have it, keep their asthma from being under control? There is no simple answer, but much more information is now known about those factors that contribute to asthma, some of which are changeable by the affected individual and family, some not.

Secondhand Smoke

Irritants such as tobacco smoke can aggravate asthma. Although tobacco use overall is on a decline, a core of smokers clings to the habit. About 1 in every 4 Americans smoke, so secondhand exposure by children from a smoking parent is likely a common occurrence.

Mothers who smoke are more likely to have babies who wheeze, have breathing difficulties, and need to be hospitalized. Children who come from homes where people smoke make more than twice as many emergency hospital visits as children who are not exposed to smoke. Overall, youngsters whose parents smoke have more frequent severe asthma attacks and need higher doses of asthma medications. Children exposed to tobacco smoke are also at increased risk for ear infections, bronchitis, pneumonia, and cough.

An American Lung Association study found that children's wheezing bouts could be reduced by 20% if parents did not smoke in the family home. Smoking is a major health risk, but there are steps that you can take to reduce your child's exposure to smoke. Don't allow anyone to smoke in your home or car. If someone in your family still smokes, despite everything that's known about the harm the habit causes, urge him to get help to quit. Research shows that a combination of medication or nicotine replacement plus counseling by a trained counselor is the most effective way to quit smoking. Many hospitals and American Lung Association chapters offer programs that can help. A "Dear Smoker" letter from your child's doctor may help persuade a smoking family member to try quitting for the sake of the child.

Air Quality

Air pollution has been linked to worsening of asthma symptoms and the rate of hospital admissions for asthma. Children with asthma who live in inner-city neighborhoods often have more respiratory problems because of bad air quality in these urban areas. Studies have shown that motor vehicle exhaust and changes in air pollution levels are closely associated with asthma symptoms and missed school days for children living in these areas. However, while it is easy to blame pollution for the increasing number of people with asthma, the fact is that the air we breathe today, in general, is much better than 30 years ago, largely because of the various Clean Air Acts passed by Congress that have improved air quality standards. So the answer to the question as to why asthma is on the rise is complicated and likely due to a combination of factors, not simply one.

The sensible approach to air pollution is to check air quality reports in weather forecasts and on the Internet or in the newspaper. When the air quality is bad, follow your pediatrician's recommendations about keeping your child indoors, monitoring breathing, and being extra careful that she take her asthma medications as prescribed. If possible, run an air conditioner during hot weather and on ozone-alert days.

Environmental Triggers

If you have asthma, it is important to identify what things in your environment might trigger your asthma. Here are some common asthma triggers.

- Tobacco smoke
- Strong odors and other irritants such as room deodorizers, perfumes, scented candles, incense, cleaning solutions, and wood-burning stoves
- Allergies such as dust mites, pet dander, molds, pollens, cockroach, and pests
- Air pollution
- Viral and bacterial infections
- Exercise or exposure to cold, dry air
- Changes in weather such as sudden temperature change

Genetic Influences

Surveys repeatedly show that asthma is much more prevalent among African Americans than whites. African Americans are hospitalized for asthma almost 3 times as often as whites, and their rate of fatal asthma attacks is also almost triple that of whites.

Although Puerto Rican children living in New York, NY, have one of the highest rates of asthma in the United States, similar rates are not seen in all children of Hispanic origin. For example, asthma is actually a little less common among Mexican American children living in the southwestern states as compared with whites.

In studying genetic patterns among African Americans, whites, and Hispanics with asthma, researchers have found several asthma-susceptibility genes linked to chromosomal regions that are unique to one or another of the ethnic groups. Much more remains to be done in this area, but the findings to date suggest that genes and environmental influences may play different roles in the various groups. The results may also eventually help to explain why the number of cases and the severity of asthma differ widely among the various segments of the population. In time, information from gene studies may make it possible to draw up guidelines for better ways to treat asthma in different population groups.

Boys Versus Girls

Up to age 14 years, boys with asthma outnumber girls with asthma by a ratio of nearly 2:1. Although asthma occurs more frequently in boys, there is no difference in the severity of asthma between boys and girls, and for now, asthma is treated the same way regardless of gender. Perhaps future studies on the causes of asthma may eventually suggest that different approaches should be taken. There are probably many reasons for the gender discrepancy seen in childhood asthma and it may take many years before we find out what they are. However, airway size may be one contributing factor. Young boys, on average, have smaller lungs relative to body size than girls. This changes as boys grow bigger, so boys may have fewer asthma symptoms after puberty starts. Girls, on the other hand, may have more asthma symptoms around puberty, possibly related to female hormones. Boys also tend to have more respiratory infections than girls do, and viral respiratory infections are among the main triggers for asthma. As children grow up, the number of boys and girls with asthma evens out.

Overweight

The rise in asthma cases is paralleled by a corresponding rise in obesity and excess weight among American children. Although there isn't a proven cause and effect between asthma and obesity, children who are overweight have a higher rate of asthma than those whose weight is within the healthy range for their height. A recent study showed that obese children were 77% more likely to have asthma. Asthma can also be more difficult to control in children who are overweight. If you are obese and have asthma, you are more likely to have severe asthma, require higher doses of asthma medicines, and have more frequent ED visits for asthma attacks. Obesity can affect lung growth, resulting in smaller lungs and possible permanent changes in lung function.

Despite widespread efforts to educate families about healthy eating, Americans of all ages are getting heavier, and it is estimated that obesity affects 61 million Americans. At least 1 American child in 4 is overweight or at risk. Too much food and too little activity are the obvious causes. Many children spend long hours every day in passive entertainment such as TV or video viewing and playing computer games. Families often rely on fast and convenience foods, which are higher in fat and calories than home-cooked meals.

Provide healthy meals and snacks for your child, emphasizing whole grains, vegetables, and fruits. Encourage her to stay in shape with regular, moderate exercise. If she doesn't like to exercise alone, join her in a daily walk; it will be good for both of you. Children with asthma who keep fit seem to have better control of their disease. The American Academy of Pediatrics recommends limiting time in front of the TV to 1 to 2 hours a day, and that includes time spent playing computer and video games for entertainment. Starting an exercise program and a weight-reduction program may lead to better asthma control and help improve overall quality of life.

Income Versus Outcome

Some children with asthma live in families with low income, and it is known that there is a direct link between the level of income and the bad outcomes of asthma in these children. There are many possible reasons as to why poverty is associated with worse outcomes. Many low-income families don't have enough information about the asthma treatments available to their children. Also, too many fall outside the reach of medical coverage. Because they lack regular pediatric care, they tend to rely on hospital EDs for their basic health services. To save money, families may skimp on medications and lose control of their child's asthma and the underlying airway inflammation that drives asthma. When symptoms occur, a family may delay taking a child to the ED until she is having serious trouble breathing, making it harder for medications to help, so that a hospital admission ends up being required.

Doctors who treat children with asthma warn that lack of regular asthma care and a delay in recognition of worsening asthma symptoms can be deadly. Using a practical, educational approach, many hospitals now provide outreach services to improve asthma care. Trained asthma counselors assist families in decreasing asthma triggers from their homes and adopting preventive measures for long-term asthma control, instead of putting out fires with emergency visits.

A priority in most asthma education programs is helping families with asthma accept the importance of daily control and recognize the early warning signs that treatment needs to be started or stepped up. Such programs have been successful in weaning many families from total dependence on emergency services to self-directed management and long-term control of asthma.

Environmental Measures to Get Rid of Allergy Triggers

Although substandard housing and crowded living conditions are sometimes blamed for the high rate of asthma among inner-city dwellers, asthma is also common among those who live in newly constructed, well-insulated homes and work in up-to-date school or office buildings. Modern construction materials tend to trap allergens and indoor pollutants in a way that drafty little houses on the prairie never did. However, it would be a mistake to try to manage asthma by dropping out of school or living in log cabins.

Letting in Air

When it comes to ventilating your home, and letting air in, you may find yourself in a quandary if you or your child suffers from seasonal pollen allergies. This is because keeping windows and doors open can allow airborne pollens to enter into the home. If you want to open doors and windows to let in outside air, wait until after mid-morning because pollen counts are highest, on average, between 5:00 and 10:00 am. When pollen counts are high it may be a good idea to limit your child's outdoor activities. After playing outside, have your child shower and wash his hair. Pollen collects on the skin and hair and if not washed off, can rub off on bedclothes and trigger asthma at night. Asthma and allergy experts recommend the use of central air-conditioning as a compromise, when the family budget allows. An air conditioner is also a form of air filtration, which can be useful during the pollen season. With an air conditioner running, pollens are filtered out and the air in your home stays drier, which also helps to reduce the mite and mold population. Most TV and radio stations, as well as newspapers, will report seasonal pollen counts in your area. You can also monitor pollen counts on the Internet through pollen counting stations such as the National Allergy Bureau at www.aaaai.org/nab.

What to Look for in an Air Filtration System

Some studies show that air filtration systems help those with asthma; others don't show any significant improvement in symptoms. If you decide to use an air filtration system, you will need to choose between a central and a portable unit. Central units are convenient in that all rooms are supplied with filtered air when the unit is on. However, portable room units have certain advantages over central ones, including

- They usually cost less.
- They can be moved from room to room as your child moves about.
- They can be taken along if the family vacates the home, whereas a central unit may be difficult to remove.
- They can be taken along on vacation or when your child is staying away from home.

If you decide on a portable unit, make sure its capacity is large enough to clean the room in which you intend to use it. Also know that the windows and door of the room where the air purifier is running need to be closed during the time of operation for the filtration to be effective.

An air filtration unit should carry the following information on its sales tag:

- CFM: The rate of *cubic feet per minute* shows how much air the unit cleans per minute. The larger the CFM rating, the more air cleaned per minute.
- RSP: *Respirable* (breathable) *size particle;* the unit should filter out particles measured at 0.03 μm and larger, which is the range likely to settle in the lungs.
- CADR: *Clean air delivery rate* shows the volume of air that moves through and is cleaned by the filtration system. A system with a higher CADR number will keep the air cleaner than one with a lower CADR number, no matter what size room.
- Warranty: Most manufacturers of high-quality units offer a lifetime warranty for central units and replaceable filters for portable units.

Forced-air heating and ventilation ducts that are part of a heating, ventilation, and air-conditioning (HVAC) system can be sources of irritants such as dust and allergens; in an ideal world, all children with asthma would live in homes fitted with baseboard heating systems or steam radiators, which don't blow warm air and dust through vents. However, because it's not often possible to replace a heating or air-conditioning system, the best you can do is take steps to reduce the entry of asthma triggers. For example, you could fit the HVAC system with a high-quality air filter, and clean and change the filter regularly. You could also run a high-efficiency particulate air (HEPA) cleaner in a room with the doors and windows shut. Keep in mind, however, that neither these nor other precautionary measures to reduce asthma triggers have been scientifically proven as effective for everyone with asthma.

Dust Mites

Among the most common asthma triggers in homes are dust mites. Dust mites live primarily in our bedding, carpet, and upholstered furnishings and they grow more when the indoor humidity is high. There are ways that you can reduce the dust mite levels in your home, although there is no way to completely eliminate them no matter how clean you try to keep your home. Encasing pillows, mattresses, and box springs in special allergen-proof zippered fabric or plastic covers can help. Bedding should be washed in hot water once weekly. If possible, remove wall-to-wall carpeting and use area throw rugs that can be washed on a regular basis. Keep indoor humidity low by using air-conditioning and a dehumidifier in particularly damp areas of the home such as a basement. Humidifiers are not recommended for people with dust mite allergy. Frequent wet mopping of hard floors or vacuuming of carpet can help to reduce dust mite levels as well. However, know that using a vacuum cleaner can sometimes stir up as much dust as it removes. If cost permits, consider purchasing special allergy vacuum cleaner bags that are double-walled and have smaller openings to prevent dust from escaping into the air. An alternative but more expensive approach is to invest in a vacuum cleaner that is equipped with a HEPA filter.

As an alternative, you may try acaricides (mite killers), cleaners, and other products made with tannic acid or benzyl benzoate, available through allergy product retailers and catalogs (see Appendix C). Applied regularly to carpets and upholstered furniture, they can help to keep down the dust mite allergen load.

Molds

Try to control molds in your home by making conditions uncomfortable for them. Kill off mildew stains as soon as you find them. Although molds can grow almost anywhere, areas where you're likely to find heavy growths are places where moisture gathers and condenses—bathroom walls and fixtures, shower curtains, under-sink cupboards in bathrooms and kitchens, basement walls and floors, and window frames. Adequate dehumidification and fixing leaky areas in basements and bathrooms helps reduce new mold growth. In a family with asthma, it may not be a good idea to bring the outdoors indoors by cultivating plants in pots. Molds that grow in the soil may be among your child's allergy asthma triggers.

Sponge moldy areas with a fungicide cleaner or a mixture of 1 part chlorine bleach and 10 parts water. Throw away rugs and fabrics that have water damage or smell musty. Get rid of carpets and upholstered furniture in the basement and bathrooms, where high humidity generally favors mold growth. To clean a mildewed plastic or vinyl shower curtain, machine wash it along with several towels in hot water with a cup of bleach. Hang it back in the shower to drip dry (vinyl and plastic can't go into the clothes dryer).

Keep the indoor humidity level low and avoid using humidifiers. Use a dehumidifier where needed to get rid of dampness. As a bonus, lowering the humidity of your home to below 50%, a level that's uncomfortable for molds, will also discourage dust mites. Like molds, mites thrive in warm, moist environments. If you have air-conditioning, keep it running to dry out the air. Clean air conditioner filters regularly to remove accumulated molds and other contaminants. To get rid of mold in closets, thoroughly clean the closet and, if possible, leave a 100-watt lightbulb on day and night to raise the temperature and dry the air.

Mold can be problematic in damp areas of the home such as basements, bathrooms, or any areas where water leakage has occurred. You should repair leaking pipes promptly. Wet carpeting should be removed or thoroughly dried as quickly as possible. Dehumidifiers in basements and other damp areas can help, but remember to empty them and clean the units regularly to prevent mold growth. If possible, you should avoid placing carpet in areas of the home prone to dampness and moisture. Exhaust fans are recommended in bathrooms and kitchens to ensure adequate ventilation. If there is extensive mold in the home, a professional service may be needed.

Avoiding Airborne Irritants

Try to keep your home free of the many irritating odors and volatile products that can act as triggers for asthma. Stay alert for irritants that may trigger your child's asthma in friends' or relatives' homes, stores, and public areas.

- Avoid smoke from wood fires and barbecues.
- Watch out for mothballs, room deodorizers, and ammonia-based cleaning products. Avoid using these in the home.
- Stay away from perfume departments and shops that carry highly perfumed goods such as candles or incense.
- Buy unscented tissues, toilet paper, laundry detergents, soaps, and other household supplies.

Pets

Unfortunately there are no real hypoallergenic cats or dogs, so if you or your child are pet allergic, the best way to manage this is avoidance. This means not getting a pet to which your child is allergic. If you already have a pet, keeping the animal outdoors is only a partial solution, as the pet allergen can still get inside the home. The best recommendation is to find another good home for the pet and thoroughly clean the home after the pet has been removed. If you cannot avoid exposure, you should definitely try to minimize contact with the pet. Don't let the pet sleep on your child's bed or even get in to the bedroom. Vacuum often and replace carpet with hardwood flooring, tile, or linoleum if possible. A HEPA air cleaner may help to reduce pet allergen levels in the air.

Pests: Cockroach, Mouse, and Rat

Cockroach and pest allergy are major triggers for asthma in children who live in inner-city neighborhoods, particularly in multifamily homes and high-rise apartment buildings. Recent studies have shown that children with mouse allergy, who are exposed to high levels of mouse allergen in their home, have more frequent ED visits and hospitalizations. High levels of cockroach, mouse, and rat allergen have been found in dust samples not only from these urban homes but also in schools and child care centers in urban areas. Dwellings with excess debris, water damage, or cracks or holes in ceilings or walls are particularly prone to cockroach and pest infestation. Pest allergens are particularly difficult to get rid of and often require a variety of elimination methods, as well as ongoing steps to prevent the pests' return.

Cockroaches can be removed by a combination of professional cleaning and baited traps. Aerosol insecticides should not be used in a home where a child with asthma lives. Instead, use sticky traps (roach motels), or sprinkle trails of boric acid powder where you can reach around water pipes and in other hard-to-get-at places where roaches nest. Boric acid, a mild germicide, is not toxic to humans, but watch that the powder isn't in places where it can irritate your child's airways. Use insecticide bombs only if you can keep your child out of your home while the bomb is active and for several hours afterward, until the rooms have been thoroughly aired and the odor is completely gone. Removing clutter and trash from the home, cleaning the kitchen well after meals, keeping food in closed containers, and filling in cracks or crevices are also recommended. High-efficiency particulate air filters have also been shown to reduce cockroach allergen levels.

For removing mouse allergen, a combination of filling in holes and cracks, vacuuming, cleaning, baited traps, and pesticides can help. These activities to reduce pest allergen levels in the home can decrease wheezing, nighttime and daytime asthma symptoms, and missed days from school.

For families like the Gibbons, paying attention to asthma triggers in the home can have great return on one's efforts. Making the right changes in Adam's environment, along with doing the other important parts of an asthma management program (knowing about the disease itself, recognizing asthma warning signs, knowing what medicines to take and when and how to take them), the Gibbons now feel like they have control of Adam's disease, rather than his disease controlling the family.

Chapter 13

Asthma Care: More Than Medication

*W*hen your child is young, asthma prevention and treatment are your responsibility. But as a child matures, he needs opportunities to assume increasing responsibility for managing his asthma. What he learns, as time goes on, is that he can control his asthma and not be controlled by it. For the young child with asthma, properly educating and preparing caregivers for asthma and asthma treatment will help parents feel comfortable when leaving the child with someone other than themselves. Finally, common problems that can interfere with good asthma management (eg, adolescent risk-taking behavior, divorced parents, concern about medication addiction) need to be addressed early on, using the child's doctor as a resource and a sounding board.

Jason's parents remind him many times to take the daily inhaled corticosteroid his doctor prescribed. But Jason, a typical teenager, just isn't interested. When he feels symptoms coming on, he relies on his albuterol inhaler. In time, Jason's parents quit nagging him about the inhaled corticosteroid because he seems to get by. Once in a while, however, he leaves home without checking that his albuterol spray is in his pocket. Right away, he begins to feel anxious and his palms get sweaty; obviously, he heavily relies on the albuterol.

A severe attack at Halloween finally convinces Jason that his parents and doctor have been right all along about preventive medications. While he is at a friend's party, he begins to have asthma symptoms that are not relieved by his albuterol inhaler. He continues trying it, hoping the medicine will kick in, but it never does. Jason has heard about people having severe attacks and even dying from their asthma, but he thinks that this is something that happens to other people, not him. As his breathing becomes more labored, it dawns on Jason's friends that the wheezing and blue color are not part of his Halloween disguise. They take him to the emergency department. Jason has to spend 4 days in the hospital, including 24 hours in the intensive care unit (ICU) for intensive asthma therapy. After this experience, Jason and his parents are determined to make sure he never has another one like it. Jason begins to take his daily controller medication, makes sure he always has refills at the pharmacy, and monitors his asthma carefully. It isn't really hard for Jason to stay on his treatment program; all it takes is a few minutes each morning and night.

The whole family has learned how important it is to take a preventive approach by controlling Jason's bronchial inflammation with daily medication.

Five Degrees of Asthma Management

The following 5 steps of asthma management were adapted from a guide developed by Thomas Plaut, MD, a physician and author who has helped thousands of children and adults control their asthma. The 5 stages are

Stage 1: No Knowledge
• Cannot recognize an asthma episode.
• Knows nothing about asthma medications.

Stage 2: Beginner
• Can recognize an asthma episode but cannot judge severity.
• Needs help in deciding when to start medication.
• Cannot communicate clearly with doctor or nurse by phone.

Stage 3: Intermediate
• Can handle an episode well with doctor's help.
• Knows how to judge severity of an episode (uses a peak flow meter, if prescribed).
• Knows when to start medications.
• Can communicate clearly with doctor or nurse by phone.
• Has made some environmental changes to reduce asthma triggers.

Stage 4: Advanced
• Has good understanding of asthma signs, triggers, and treatments.
• Skillfully analyzes symptoms; knows when to start and stop medications (understands how to act on a peak flow reading, if one being used).
• Can handle most episodes safely at home or elsewhere without consulting doctor or nurse.
• Has made major environmental changes to reduce triggers.

Stage 5: Expert
• Fully understands asthma symptoms, triggers, and medications.
• Can accurately judge symptoms and knows when to seek help. Understands course and pattern of episodes.
• Can assess episodes and use this information to discuss ways to improve treatment.
• Needs doctor's help only if symptoms are unusually severe.
• Reviews treatment with doctor at regular 3- to 12-month intervals.

Adapted from Plaut T. *One Minute Asthma: What You Need to Know.* 8th ed. Amherst, MA: Pedipress Inc; 2008

Jason's need for the rapid-relief medication that he used to live off drops way down as he follows through with the daily treatment plan. Jason no longer feels nervous if he leaves home without his albuterol inhaler. He finds that he can now keep up with the other kids in the pickup basketball games he loves to play after school. After a while, his parents don't need to check on whether he takes his medication. Jason has grown up a lot; he has become much more responsible for his asthma care and much less dependent on his parents. And whenever he is tempted to skip a treatment, a flashback to his time in the ICU renews his determination to stay out of the hospital.

. . . .

$\mathcal{Y}$ou, as the parent, are totally responsible for the management of your child's asthma when she is very young. However, in ideal circumstances, your child would progress steadily upward from stage 1 (no knowledge), reaching stage 5 (expert) by her late teens (see "Five Degrees of Asthma Management" on page 136). In reality, of course, the ability to take charge of asthma management is subject to many variables, including each person's emotional maturity and organizational skills. There are plenty of young adolescents who are willing and able to assume responsibility for their own asthma treatment. By contrast, there will always be some rebellious teenagers and emotionally immature adults who may never achieve good control because they refuse to face facts and accept the need for a systematic approach to the disease.

As the parent of a child with asthma, you will progress along with your child, starting with total responsibility for all aspects of care and prevention and gradually handing over more of the treatment package. With asthma care, as with other aspects of your child's drive toward independence, you may sometimes find it difficult to give her the freedom she wants. Or your child may progress in stops and starts, alternately demanding more responsibility than she can handle and regressing to clinging and overdependence for a while. It is important to recognize that this fluctuating behavior is typical for adolescents, and that turning asthma care into a source of conflict between parent and teenager should be avoided. Furthermore, even a teenager who is responsible needs ongoing parental guidance, including in asthma care.

As noted, during adolescence, asthma management can be complicated by various emotional conflicts—feelings of invincibility, rebelliousness, and risk-taking, among others. While it may sometimes be difficult, keep the lines of communication open, and help the adolescent gain independence and assume responsibility for her asthma management. If tensions and conflicts threaten to disrupt your youngster's asthma treatment, ask your pediatrician for some unbiased advice or perhaps for a referral to an experienced family counselor. Asthma support groups provide opportunities for parents and children with asthma to learn that others share their difficulties. Those who take part may have practical suggestions for heading off trouble or improving a deteriorating situation. Ask your pediatrician to put you in touch with a local support group, or contact a national organization such as the Asthma and Allergy Foundation of America or the American Lung Association, which can suggest resources in your area; see Appendix B for national resources.

Communication Among Family Members

Although one family member's asthma may affect everyone in the family one way or another, it shouldn't be allowed to limit the family's activities. If a sibling feels she's being neglected for the sake of another with asthma, she's likely to develop a smoldering resentment that may lead to deep emotional rifts.

Clear communication helps family members of every generation, grandparents to toddlers, understand how asthma occurs and why medications and environmental measures are required to keep it under control. Booklets, the child's written treatment plan, and videos are useful educational tools. (See Appendix B.) Family members, when properly informed, become sensitive to the warning signs of asthma and can recognize when the child with asthma needs help. When all family members understand what's happening and how to manage the situation, they are less likely to fall into 1 of the 2 main pitfalls—panicking when symptoms threaten, or ignoring worsening symptoms until the child with asthma is in trouble and can't breathe.

Staying With the Treatment Program

Most severe asthma attacks can be prevented if those with asthma get the proper diagnosis and follow their treatment plan. When people with asthma wind up in emergency care, it's easy to put the blame on poverty, lack of information, and problems of access to health services. But this doesn't explain why too many children and adults with asthma keep on having bouts of severe breathing troubles even after effective treatment programs have been prescribed.

Asthma treatment can be complicated. A child with asthma has to follow many different instructions. Not only does he have to keep in mind which medications and how much of them to take, but he also has to know how to use inhalers and other medication delivery devices, avoid asthma triggers as much as possible, and recognize when acute symptoms threaten so he can seek help at once.

None of this is easy. Generally speaking, the fewer medications and the fewer daily doses a youngster has to take, the more likely he is to do so. However, children, particularly adolescents, tend to resist any medical treatment program in the following circumstances, all of which are typical of asthma treatment:

- When treatment must go on for a long time—perhaps even indefinitely
- When medication is used to prevent the onset of symptoms, rather than to get rid of symptoms already present
- When symptoms don't always follow right away if a dose of medication is skipped

This is why some youngsters with asthma have difficulty following a treatment plan. They accept the need for using their asthma medications consistently only after severe symptoms have recurred repeatedly when treatment has been neglected.

Many other factors interfere with the success of asthma treatment. For example, family members may not encourage the child with asthma to follow his treatment plan if the medications are expensive or there is concern about side effects (see Chapter 11, page 110). If the child isn't actually wheezing or having trouble breathing, the family may think that medications aren't needed. Families who tend to seek advice from alternative health prac-titioners (See Chapter 11, page 120) are sometimes resistant to the idea of using medica-tions, especially preventive medications for long-term asthma control when the child is not having symptoms.

The severity of the illness plays a key role; surveys have shown that youngsters with moder-ate asthma are more likely to follow their pediatricians' instructions than those with mild or severe asthma. In the case of mild asthma, they may think that the condition isn't serious enough to warrant treatment. In the case of severe asthma, perhaps they are trying to deny that the disease is present, or they may become discouraged and feel that medications don't help. Whatever the case may be, lack of treatment can lead to symptoms and disability.

Concerns About Medication Dependence

Some people worry that their child will become dependent on, or even addicted to, asthma medications if she takes them daily over an extended period. Medications for asthma are different from the types of drugs that cause addiction. Furthermore, doctors prescribe the lowest dose level and the least frequent schedule of dosing, preferring to give only enough medication to ensure a good treatment effect while keeping side effects to a low level. If your child's asthma is under poor control, your doctor may start treatment at a higher dose level to bring asthma under control, then decrease the medication to a low, maintenance level once your child is comfortable with the treatment program.

With the medications and delivery devices currently available for asthma treatment, you don't need to worry about medication dependence or addiction. If your child's doctor sees that the youngster tends to overuse a particular medication, like her quick-relief inhaler, it's usually a signal that asthma is not under proper control, not a sign of addiction. What it means is that the treatment plan needs to be revised.

What Child Care Providers Need to Know

It's not unusual for parents of children with asthma to feel apprehensive about leaving their child in someone else's care. On top of all the unexpected mishaps that can occur even in the best-run homes, parents worry that their child with asthma will have sudden, severe symptoms and the caregiver won't know how to take action in time.

To keep asthma in perspective, head off clinging, and maintain healthy family relationships, it's important to get used to leaving your child in the care of a reliable caregiver. You can feel confident leaving your child for a break as long as you've prepared the child and equipped the caregiver with everything needed, including emergency phone numbers. Involve your child in the process; he'll enjoy taking responsibility for educating his care-giver about asthma.

Even if your caregiver claims to know about asthma, get hold of an educational video and watch it with your caregiver to make sure up-to-date information is available. Review your child's usual asthma triggers and emphasize the importance of avoiding triggers when possible. Write down the 4 major signs of asthma—coughing, wheezing, fast breathing, and the chest being sucked in on each breath. Review your written instructions about what to do in case your child has any or all of the symptoms while you're gone. If your child uses a peak flow meter, demonstrate how to work the device and use it to let the caregiver know when to call for help, if necessary.

Give the caregiver clearly written information about quick-relief medications—their names, doses, how each medication is given, what the desired effects are and how soon to expect them, and side effects. Review your child's treatment plan with the caregiver and write down all instructions. In leaving the usual emergency phone numbers and the number where you can be reached, provide the number of a trusted friend or neighbor as a backup, and let this person know when you're leaving and when you intend to return.

Asthma Care in Divorced Families

When a child divides her time between divorced or separated parents, both parents need to stay fully informed about asthma and the medications used in their child's treatment. Each household should have a complete set of the child's asthma medications and the written treatment plan, regularly updated. To keep communication channels open as much as possible, both former partners (along with new partners who share in the responsibility for the child) should try to be present together at their child's visits to the doctor's office. If this is not possible, ask for duplicate copies of materials that are given (eg, updated asthma action plans, educational materials) and set aside a few minutes of time to go over the materials together.

One parent usually spends more time with the child day to day. This parent may be more attuned to the condition and have more opportunities for learning about asthma. However, this information should be shared for the benefit of the child. If ex-spouses have difficulty communicating with each other, their child's pediatrician can provide straightforward information to both sides and help them keep the youngster's well-being in perspective.

Divorced parents sometimes tend to act out anger and resentment toward the ex-partner, using their child's asthma as a reason or excuse. This is unacceptable and must be avoided. Differences of opinion may arise between ex-partners over the child's need for medication, the importance of avoiding certain allergy triggers, and activities that are suitable for the child. One parent may accuse the other of being overprotective or too casual with regard to the amount of attention paid to asthma symptoms and prevention. To avoid hostility, which could cause severe emotional stress to the child, parents must try to deal with any differences of opinion in an open and communicative way. Putting the child or the child's doctor between warring parents is not fair to the child or the doctor and often puts the child's health at risk. If you have difficulty discussing your child's asthma care or any other aspects of her care, ask your pediatrician to refer you to an experienced counselor who may be able to suggest strategies for working out an acceptable compromise.

APPENDIXES

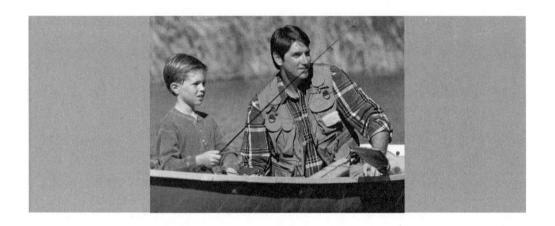

Appendix A

Hidden Food Allergens

Potentially allergenic foods may be used in natural or processed form for preparing commercial foods. Allergic children (when old enough) and their parents must read all food labels thoroughly to identify clear and hidden food allergens. Following are some terms to watch for (all tables adapted from "'Hidden' Allergens in Foods," by Harris A. Steinman, MBChB, *Journal of Allergy and Clinical Immunology*, Vol 98, p 241–250, published by Mosby-Year Book Inc.):

Labels That May Indicate Presence of Egg Protein

Albumin	Globulin	Ovomucoid
Binder	Lecithin	Ovovitellin
Coagulant	Livetin	Powdered egg
Egg white	Lysozyme	Vitellin
Egg yolk/yellow	Ovalbumin	Whole egg
Emulsifier	Ovomucin	

Foods That May Contain Egg Protein

Baked goods (most, except some breads)	Hollandaise sauce	Puddings
Baking mixes	Ice cream	Salad dressings (creamy)
Batters	Lemon curd	Sherbets
Béarnaise sauce	Macaroni	Souffles
Bouillon (in restaurants to clear it)	Malted cocoa drinks (eg, Ovaltine, Ovamalt)	Soups
Breakfast cereals	Marshmallows	Spaghetti
Cake flours	Mayonnaise	Sweets (eg, fondant creams, truffles, marshmallows)
Candy (see Sweets)	Meringues	Tartar sauce
Cookies	Muffins	Turkish delight
Creamy fillings	Noodles (egg)	Waffles
Custard	Omelets	Wines (if cleared with egg white)
Egg noodles	Pancakes	
Eggnog	Processed meat products (eg, bologna, meat loaf, meatballs, sausages)	
French toast		

Labels That May Indicate the Presence of Milk Protein

Artificial butter flavor	Dried milk	Pasteurized milk
Butter	Dry milk solids	Rennet casein
Butterfat	Fully cream milk powder	Skim milk powder
Buttermilk solids	High-protein flavoring	Solids
Caramel color	Lactalbumin	Sour cream (or solids)
Caramel flavoring	Lactalbumin phosphate	Sour milk solids
Casein	Lactose	Whey
Caseinate	Milk	Whey powder
Cheese	Milk derivative	Whey protein concentrate
Cream curds	Milk protein	Yogurt
"De-lactosed" whey	Milk solids	
Demineralized whey	Natural flavoring	

Foods That May Contain Milk Protein

Batter-fried foods	Custard	Packaged soups
Biscuits	Fish in batter	Pies
Bread	Gravies and gravy mixes	Puddings
Breakfast cereals	Ice cream (and "non-milk" fat)	Rusks
Cakes	Imitation sour cream	Sausages
Canned soups	Instant mashed potatoes	Sherbet
Chocolate	Margarine	Soy cheese
Cookies	Muesli	Soup mixes
Cream sauces	Muffins	Sweets
Cream soups	Other baked goods	Vegetarian cheese

Labels That May Indicate the Presence of Soy Protein

Bulking agent	Protein	Stabilizer
Carob	Protein extender	Starch
Emulsifier	Soy flour	Textured vegetable protein
Guar gum	Soy nuts	(TVP)
Gum arabic	Soy panthenol	Thickener
Hydrolyzed vegetable protein (HVP)	Soy protein	Tofu
	Soy protein isolate or concentrate	Vegetable broth
Lecithin[a]	Soy sauce	Vegetable gum
Miso	Soybean	Vegetable starch
Monosodium glutamate (MSG)[b]	Soybean oil	

[a]Mostly produced from soy but may be manufactured from egg.
[b]Sometimes produced from soy or wheat but now mostly by synthetic means.

Foods That May Contain Soy Protein

Baby foods
Bakery goods[a]
Black pudding
Bread (especially high-
    protein bread)[a]
Breakfast cereals (some)
Burger patties
Butter substitutes
Cakes
Candy
Canned meat or fish in
    sauces[a]
Canned or packaged
    soups[a]
Canned tuna
Cheese (artificial) made
    from soybeans[a]
Chinese food
Chocolates (cream centers)

Cookies
Cooking oils
Crackers
Desserts
Gravy (sauce) powders
Hamburger patties
Hot dogs
Hydrolyzed vegetable
    protein (may be wheat)
Ice cream
Infant formula (including
    cow's-milk formula)
Liquid meal replacers
Margarine
Meat products (eg, sausages,
    pastes, Vienna sausages
    [wieners])
Muesli
Pies (meat or other)[a]

Powdered meal replacers
Salad dressings
Sauces (eg, Worcestershire,
    sweet and sour, HP, teriyaki)
Seasoned salt
Shortenings
Snack bars
Soups
Soy pasta products
Soy sauce
Soy sprouts (Chinese restaurants)
Soybeans
Stews (commercial)
Stock cubes (bouillon cubes)
Tofu
Tofutti
TV dinners

[a]May be present because of soya in the flour used.

Other Sources of Contact With Soy

Adhesives
Blankets
Body lotions and creams
Dog food
Enamel paints

Fabric finishes
Fabrics
Fertilizers
Flooring materials
Lubricants

Nitroglycerin
Paper
Printing inks
Soaps

Labels That May Indicate the Presence of Wheat Protein

All-purpose flour	Hard durum flour	Vegetable gum[a]
Bleached flour	High gluten flour	Vegetable starch[a]
Bulgur (cracked wheat)	High protein flour[b]	Vital gluten
Bran	Hydrolyzed vegetable protein[b]	Wheat bran
Cornstarch	Kamut	Wheat flour
Couscous	Miller's bran	Wheat germ
Durum wheat	Modified food starch[a]	Wheat gluten
Enriched flour	Monosodium glutamate (MSG)[c]	Wheat starch
Farina	Protein	White flour
Gelatinized starch[a]	Semolina	Whole wheat
(or pre-gelatinized)	Spelt	Whole wheat flour
Gluten	Starch[a]	
Graham flour	Unbleached flour	

[a]May indicate the presence of soy protein or may be manufactured from cassava (tapioca), maize, or rice.
[b]Sometimes produced from soy or wheat but now mostly by synthetic means.
[c]May be soy.

Foods That May Contain Wheat

Alcoholic Beverages
Ale (made from grain
  alcohol)
Beer
Bourbon
Whiskey
Wine

Baked Goods
Baking mixes
Barley bread and drinks
Battered foods
Biscuit breads (including
  rye bread)
Bouillon cubes
Breaded meats
Breaded vegetables
Breakfast cereals

Cakes
Candy or chocolate candy
Canned processed meat
Cereal grains
Cookies
Couscous
Crackers
Gravy
Hot dogs
Ice cream
Ice cream cones
Luncheon meats
Licorice
Macaroni
Malt
Malted milks (eg, Horlicks)
Milk shakes

Noodle products
Pasta (noodles, spaghetti,
  macaroni)
Pepper (compound or
  powdered flour filler)
Pies
Processed meats
Sausage
Semolina
Snack foods
Spaghetti
Soup mixes
Soups
Soy sauce
Tablets

Foods That May Contain Peanut or Peanut Oil

Baked goods	Chinese dishes	Pastry
Baking mixes	Chocolate	Peanut butter
Battered foods	Cookies	Satay sauce and dishes
Biscuits	Egg rolls	Soups
Breakfast cereals	Ice cream	Sweets
Candy	Margarine	Thai dishes
Cereal-based products	Marzipan	Vegetable fat
Chili	Milk formula	Vegetable oil

Most near-fatal and fatal allergic reactions to food happen when people are eating away from home. A person who is highly allergic should wear a medical ID bracelet or tag and carry an epinephrine (adrenaline) autoinjector at all times. If a family member is severely allergic, it's probably safest to avoid all commercially processed foods unless you are certain that they are made and packaged by a reliable manufacturer. The Food Allergy & Anaphylaxis Network (see Appendix B) regularly updates information on its Web site (www.foodallergy.org) about foods commonly associated with allergies.

Appendix B

Allergy and Asthma Resources

Organizations

Allergy & Asthma Network Mothers of Asthmatics
8201 Greensboro Dr, Suite 300
McLean, VA 22102
800/878-4403
www.aanma.org

American Academy of Allergy, Asthma & Immunology
555 E Wells St, Suite 1100
Milwaukee, WI 53202-3823
414/272-6071
www.aaaai.org

American Academy of Pediatrics
141 Northwest Point Blvd
Elk Grove Village, IL 60007-1019
847/434-4000
www.aap.org

American Association for Respiratory Care
9425 N MacArthur Blvd, Suite 100
Irving, TX 75063-4706
972/243-2272
www.aarc.org

American College of Allergy, Asthma & Immunology
85 W Algonquin Rd, Suite 550
Arlington Heights, IL 60005
847/427-1200
www.acaai.org

American Lung Association
1301 Pennsylvania Ave NW, Suite 800
Washington, DC 20004
202/785-3355
www.lungusa.org

Organizations *(continued)*

Asthma and Allergy Foundation of America
8201 Corporate Dr, Suite 1000
Landover, MD 20785
800/7-ASTHMA (727-8462)
www.aafa.org

Consortium on Children's Asthma Camps
490 Concordia Ave
St Paul, MN 55103
651/227-8014
www.asthmacamps.org

Food Allergy & Anaphylaxis Network
11781 Lee Jackson Hwy, Suite 160
Fairfax, VA 22033-3309
800/929-4040
www.foodallergy.org

National Asthma Education and Prevention Program
National Heart, Lung, and Blood Institute Information Center
PO Box 30105
Bethesda, MD 20824-0105
301/592-8573
www.nhlbi.nih.gov/about/naepp

National Eczema Association
4460 Redwood Hwy, Suite 16D
San Rafael, CA 94903-1953
800/818-7546
www.nationaleczema.org

National Institute of Allergy and Infectious Diseases
Office of Communications and Government Relations
6610 Rockledge Dr, MSC 6612
Bethesda, MD 20892-6612
866/284-4107
www.niaid.nih.gov

National Jewish Health
1400 Jackson St
Denver, CO 80206
800/423-8891
www.nationaljewish.org

Publications

Asthma for Dummies
William E. Berger
Hoboken, NJ: Wiley Pub; 2004

The Harvard Medical School Guide to Taking Control of Asthma
Christopher H. Fanta, Lynda M. Cristiano, Kenan E. Haver
New York, NY: Free Press; 2003

A Parent's Guide to Asthma: How You Can Help Your Child Control Asthma
at Home, School, and Play
Nancy Sander
New York, NY: Plume; 1994
Contact Allergy & Asthma Network Mothers of Asthmatics
800/878-4403 or www.aanma.org

One-Minute Asthma: What You Need to Know
Thomas F. Plaut
8th ed. Amherst, MA: Pedipress; 2008
800/611-6081 or www.pedipress.com

Dr. Tom Plaut's Asthma Guide for People of All Ages
Thomas F. Plaut, Teresa B. Jones
Amherst, MA: Pedipress; 1999

Taming Asthma and Allergy by Controlling Your Environment: A Guide for Patients
Robert A. Wood
Baltimore, MD: Asthma and Allergy Foundation of America, Maryland Chapter; 1995
410/484-2054 or www.aafa-md.org

My House Is Killing Me! The Home Guide for Families with Allergies and Asthma
Jeffrey C. May
Baltimore, MD: Johns Hopkins University Press; 2001

Creating a Healthy Household: The Ultimate Guide for Healthier, Safer, Less-Toxic Living
Lynn Marie Bower
Bloomington, IN: Healthy House Institute; 2000

Understanding and Managing Your Child's Food Allergies
Scott H. Sicherer
Baltimore, MD: Johns Hopkins University Press; 2006

Publications *(continued)*

The Complete Peanut Allergy Handbook
Scott H. Sicherer, Terry Malloy
New York, NY: Berkley Books; 2005

Food Allergies for Dummies
Robert A. Wood, Joe Kraynak
Hoboken, NJ: Wiley Pub; 2007

Appendix C

Product Information

Allergy Asthma Technology
8145 N Austin Ave
Morton Grove, IL 60053
800/621-5545
www.allergyasthmatech.com

Allergy Control Products
22 Shelter Rock Ln
Danbury, CT 06810
800/ALLERGY (255-3749)
www.allergycontrol.com

MedicAlert Foundation
2323 Colorado Ave
Turlock, CA 95382
888/633-4298
www.medicalert.org

National Allergy Supply, Inc.
1620-D Satellite Blvd
Duluth, GA 30097
800/522-1448
www.natlallergy.com

Appendix D

Glossary

acute: Sudden; sometimes also used to mean short and relatively severe.

adenoid: A single mass of tissue in the upper part of the throat, behind the nose, that works with the tonsils to help fight germs coming in via the nose and mouth.

adrenaline: See *epinephrine.*

adrenergic: Medication that acts like epinephrine (adrenaline).

airflow: The rate at which air can be blown out of the lungs.

allergen: Substance that provokes allergy.

allergic rhinitis: A nose condition characterized by symptoms of running, itching, stuffiness, and sneezing that occur periodically or year-round.

allergist: A doctor who specializes in treating allergies.

allergy: Immune reaction to a normally harmless substance.

allergy shots: See *immunotherapy.*

alveoli: Air sacs at the ends of the smallest airways in the lungs.

anaphylaxis: Severe, total-body allergic reaction that can be fatal if not treated at once.

angioedema: Non-itchy swelling that is often but not always triggered by allergy.

antibody: Protein developed by the body in response to entry of a foreign substance (antigen), conferring immunity.

anticholinergic: Quick-relief type medication for asthma that works by blocking the passage of impulses through certain nerve pathways.

antigen: Any substance capable of inducing an immune response.

antihistamine: Medication that blocks the effects of histamine, such as itching and swelling.

anti-inflammatory: Medication that prevents or reduces inflammation.

asthma: Inflammatory airway disease in which airways are over-responsive to stimuli; symptoms can be stopped or prevented by medical and environmental measures.

atopy: Allergy.

autonomic nervous system: Nerves controlling certain functions of the heart muscle, smooth muscles (including those of the airways), skin, gastrointestinal tract, and mucous glands.

breath-activated: Device that releases medication when triggered by the user's breathing.

breathing rate: Number of breaths per minute.

bronchi, bronchus (singular): Large airways of the lungs.

bronchioles: Small airways of the lungs.

bronchiolitis: Inflammation of the small airways (bronchioles), usually caused by a viral infection.

bronchitis: Inflammation of the larger airways (bronchi) of the lungs.

bronchoconstriction: Narrowing of the airways caused by contraction of the smooth muscles (also called bronchospasm).

bronchodilator: Medication to open constricted airways of the lungs.

bronchospasm: See *bronchoconstriction.*

cartilage: Firm, flexible tissue that supports the large airways and other organs.

chemical mediator: Naturally occurring chemical (histamine, leukotriene) that plays a role in the body's immune response, which can lead to allergy and asthma symptoms.

chronic: Persistent or long-term condition (usually lasting 6 weeks or longer).

compliance: Taking medication and performing other aspects of therapy exactly as prescribed.

controlled release: Medication taken in a formulation that allows the release of predictable amounts over time (same as long-acting, slow-release, sustained-release).

controller: Term used for medication that decreases or prevents the frequency of asthma episodes, usually but not always by reducing the underlying inflammation of asthma.

corticosteroid: Synthetic form of an adrenal hormone that is used as a medication to suppress inflammation (also called steroid and cortisone).

cortisone: See *corticosteroid.*

cromolyn: Medication that prevents mast cells in the airway tissues from releasing chemical mediators that cause allergic inflammation.

croup: Barking cough caused by inflammation of the trachea and voice box.

dander: Dead skin scales.

decongestant: Medication to reduce congestion caused by fluid accumulation in tissues.

desensitization: Immunotherapy (allergy injections) to decrease or eliminate allergic response to a substance.

dry powder inhaler (DPI): A type of inhaler used for asthma where a dry powder is inhaled into the lungs.

dust mite: Microscopic arachnid, a relative of spiders and ticks, that lives around humans and in house dust, and is a frequent cause of allergies (also called mite).

eczema: Itchy flat rash (also called atopic dermatitis).

eosinophil: White blood cell involved in the immune response, especially the allergic one.

epinephrine: A hormone (also called adrenaline) produced by the adrenal glands and released in response to stress and other stimuli; a synthetic form of epinephrine is used as a medication to constrict the blood vessels and widen the airways, to help patients who have serious allergic reactions.

episode: A period when asthma symptoms occur, the ability to breathe is affected, and additional medication may be needed (also called bout or flare-up).

exercise-induced asthma: A form of asthma that is triggered by physical activity or exertion.

exhale: To breathe out.

flare-up: See *episode.*

flow monitor: Part of the holding chamber medication delivery device, which makes a warning sound if the person breathes in too fast.

food intolerance: Nonallergic adverse reaction to food, which does not involve the immune system.

gastroesophageal reflux disease (GERD): Backflow of food mixed with digestive acids from stomach into the esophagus, causing irritation that can sometimes lead to bronchoconstriction.

GERD: See *gastroesophageal reflux disease (GERD).*

hay fever: Periodic symptoms, especially of the nose and eyes, caused by pollens and other seasonal stimuli (also called seasonal allergic rhinitis).

HEPA filter/cleaner: High-efficiency particulate air filter or cleaner that removes very small particles from the air.

histamine: A chemical mediator of allergies and asthma.

hives: Itchy swellings, usually caused by allergy (also called urticaria).

holding chamber: Medication delivery device used with a metered-dose inhaler to hold the medication mist so it is easier to take, better absorbed, and more effective (it is a type of spacer).

hyperresponsive: Immune system or airways that overreact to allergy or asthma triggers.

hypersensitivity: Usually means allergy.

IgE: Immunoglobulin E; an antibody that is formed by the body in response to entry by a foreign protein that subsequently recognizes the protein as an allergen and sets off the allergic immune reaction.

immunoglobulin E: See *IgE*.

immunotherapy: Injection of small but increasing doses of a substance to bring about desensitization to that allergen (also called allergy shots or allergy desensitization).

inflammation: The body's response to a potentially injurious physical or chemical trigger, with swelling, heat, and redness caused by the mobilization of cells, fluids, and chemicals into the injured area.

inhalation device: Device that delivers medication as the person breathes in.

inhaled steroid: Synthetic hormone medication taken by breathing in that reduces existing inflammation in the airways and prevents further inflammation from developing; widely prescribed for children with persistent asthma.

inhaler: Device that allows delivery of inhaled medication into the airways.

intradermal: Into or under the skin.

irritant: A nonallergenic substance that can cause an aggravating reaction in the skin, airways, or other organ or tissues.

large airways: Air passages wider than 3 to 4 mm in diameter.

leukocyte: White blood cell (see also *lymphocyte).*

leukotriene: Chemical mediator involved in asthma and allergic inflammation.

leukotriene modifier: Medication that blocks the production or effect of leukotrienes in the airways, thus partly stopping the asthma or allergic response.

long-acting: Similar to controlled-release, slow-release, and sustained-release medications.

lung-function test: Assessment of the ability to breathe in and out, often done in asthma.

lymphocyte: Type of white blood cell.

mask: Device that fits over the nose and mouth to help in delivery and absorption of inhaled asthma medications.

mast cell: A cell that, when stimulated by an allergy or asthma trigger, releases chemicals that lead to an allergy or asthma response.

mediator: A naturally occurring chemical through which an allergy or asthma reaction takes place.

metered-dose inhaler (MDI): Device that delivers a predetermined amount of inhaled asthma medication.

monitor: Keep track of.

mouthpiece: The part of a medication delivery device that fits in a person's mouth.

mucus: Thick, protective, cleansing semiliquid produced by glands in the airways, nose, sinuses, and other organs.

nebulizer: Delivery device that converts liquid medication into a fine mist that can be inhaled.

objective sign: Event that can be seen and evaluated.

onset of effect/action: Time lapse between taking medication and feeling or seeing its effects.

ozone: A form of oxygen (O_3) that causes irritation in the airways; a component of smog or air pollution.

ozone layer: Layer of ozone in the upper atmosphere that protects the Earth's surface from the harmful effects of ultraviolet sunlight.

peak expiratory flow: Rate at which air is expelled from the lungs when your child breathes out as fast and hard as he or she can, using a peak flow meter.

peak flow meter: Device for measuring peak expiratory flow rate.

pediatrician: Doctor specializing in the health care of newborns, infants, children, adolescents, and young adults.

pollen: Fine cell grains responsible for fertilization of plants and also responsible for causing allergies.

pollutant: Impurity that contaminates air or water.

prick test: See *skin tests*.

pulmonary function test: See *lung-function test*.

quick-relief medication: Medication that acts rapidly to open constricted airways.

radioallergosorbent blood test (RAST): Measurement of IgE antibody to a specific antigen in the blood. A more contemporary term for RAST is specific IgE blood test.

RAST: See *radioallergosorbent blood test (RAST).*

rescue medicine: See *quick-relief medication.*

respirable particles: Small microscopic particles (1–5 μm in diameter) that can be inhaled into the lungs and are able to reach airways that need to be reached to treat asthma.

retraction: "Sucking in" of the skin of the chest or neck.

scratch tests: See *skin tests.*

sensitization: Process of developing an allergic response to a substance.

side effect: Undesirable or adverse effect of medication.

sign: External physical effects of an illness that can be seen and evaluated by an observer.

sinus: One of 8 air pockets, or cavities, in the bones of the front of the face.

sinusitis: Inflammation of the sinuses.

skin tests: Allergy tests in which drops of allergen extracts are allowed to seep through shallow scratches made in the skin surface.

small airways: Air passages less than 2 to 3 mm in diameter (bronchioles).

spacer: Device used with an MDI to help with coordination and to help improve delivery of medication to the lungs.

specific IgE blood test: Measurement of IgE antibody to a specific antigen in the blood. An old term for this is RAST test.

spirometer: Device used by a doctor to measure airflow into and out of the lungs.

step down: Method of asthma treatment that starts with higher medication doses to achieve control quickly, then gradually decreases medications to lowest levels required for symptom control.

step up: Method of asthma treatment that starts with a lower medication dose to achieve control, then increases the medication dose to the dose able to give symptom control.

steroid: Synthetic form of a naturally occurring hormone that can be taken by mouth or as an inhaled spray to stop inflammation and control asthma.

sustained-release: Long-acting medication.

symptoms: Physical effects of an illness that are internal or felt by the person involved (see *sign).*

tidal breathing: Normal breathing.

toxicity: Adverse effects of medication.

trachea: The windpipe, a firm tube that extends downward from the larynx and branches into the left and right bronchi.

trigger: Environmental factor that causes the body to respond with allergy or asthma symptoms.

twitchy: Description of the airways of people with asthma (eg, overreactive).

voice box: Larynx; part of the upper airways between the throat and the windpipe (trachea) where sound is produced.

wheeze: High-pitched whistle heard when air flows in and out through constricted airways.

white blood cell: Cells that work mainly to defend the body from infectious bacteria and invading allergens.

windpipe: See *trachea.*

workup: Doctor's examination and evaluation.

INDEX